The Distant Sound of Wisdom

Biblical Perspectives
on Health

Warren A. Shipton

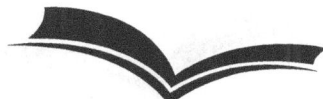

TEACH Services, Inc.
P U B L I S H I N G
www.TEACHServices.com • (800) 367-1844

Copyright © 2015 Warren A. Shipton

Copyright © 2015 TEACH Services, Inc.

ISBN-13: 978-1-4796-0563-7 (Paperback)

ISBN-13: 978-1-4796-0564-4 (ePub)

ISBN-13: 978-1-4796-0565-1 (Mobi)

Library of Congress Control Number: 2015912713

Published by

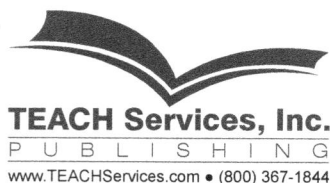

TEACH Services, Inc.
PUBLISHING
www.TEACHServices.com • (800) 367-1844

Dedicated to the memory of William Tyndale, scholar and martyr, who said of the Bible "it is called the word of life, the word of grace, the word of health, the word of redemption, the word of forgiveness, and the word of peace."

David Teems, Tyndale (Nashville, Tenn.: Thomas Nelson, 2012), 114, 115.

Contents

"Vision is not enough, it must be combined with venture.
It is not enough to stare up the steps, we must step up the stairs" (Vaclav Havel).

"That [Jesus Christ] was the true Light which gives light to every man coming into the world"
(John the Apostle).

"To see what is right, and not do it, is want of courage or of principle" (Confucius).

Foreword

Modern medicine has made tremendous advances in the past half century. Only a few hundred years ago, we humans did not know what our own anatomy was and only in the past century have we discovered some of what our organs do. Now, modern medicine can cure many diseases previously thought to be lethal, such as leprosy, malaria, tuberculosis, and even some kinds of cancer.

However, modern medicine has a dark side. Commonly used pain medicines have been found to increase the risk of heart attacks and kidney failure. Antifungal medications have been found to cause liver damage. Treatments previously used to treat cancer have been found to cause other kinds of cancer. Medicines used to prevent malaria can cause eye damage when used for long periods. You only have to look at the package insert for any prescription medicine to see all the potential problems it can cause.

Then, there are frightening public health problems. Diabetes is on the rise, not only in developed countries but in developing countries. Obesity is not just increasingly more common; it has reached epidemic proportions. Tuberculosis, once on the decline worldwide, is back on the rise in many places and often resistant to many of the previously effective drugs. Some bacteria found in hospitals have grown resistant to all known antibiotics, and this resistance is spreading rapidly to bacteria in the community. Malaria, treated for many years with quinine, is now resistant to most drugs, and some strains have been found to be resistant to all antimalarials.

Dissatisfaction with modern medicine and modern science has led many people to start using natural remedies hoping they are safer. The sale of herbal treatments and vitamins has skyrocketed, even when there is little evidence to support use of some of them. People are seeking traditional remedies worldwide in hopes of finding a better, safer treatment for their illnesses.

A difficulty comes in knowing what treatments work and what do not work. We hear conflicting reports in the press and from the medical profession. One year we hear eggs are bad for us, and a few years later we hear they are good for us. We hear sun exposure causes skin cancer, so we stay out of the sun only to develop a vitamin D deficiency, which is linked to a number of serious diseases. We hear vitamin E helps reduce the risk of heart disease, but then a few years later we find out taking vitamin E tablets does not reduce the risk of heart disease and may actually increase the risk.

Who should we believe? Where can we go to get information on how we can stay healthy in a world that seems to be getting sicker every day? If we are sick already, what can we do to get back to good health? Are there any methods that have been proven to work over the years? We do not want a method that is lauded today and condemned tomorrow. We want tried and true methods that are safe and effective.

Many of us have experienced illness during periods of stress. As a clinician, I know when examination time is at the schools because I start seeing more people coming in with colds, the flu, ulcers, and migraines. There is a link between mental and physical health. When we finish school, we may think the stress is over, but those who have worked in the world a few years know only too well stress levels only increase after school and continue to do so throughout our lives. These begin to tell on our health after a decade or two.

What can be done to prevent our mental problems from causing physical problems? Better yet, what can we do to solve our mental problems that do not involve using a harmful chemical substance such as alcohol or a prescription drug? What school of philosophy will give us peace? What coping mechanism is safe and healthy? Is there some tried and true method to give us mental health?

The author of the book you are holding has made an extensive study of a reference that answers the questions of how to have good mental and physical health. It is a reference that has been used by millions of people as not only a spiritual guide but as a guide to good mental and physical health. It is a reference that has unique qualifications to keep us healthy, but it is often taken for granted. Many people have this reference in their own homes but never realize it provides a guide for true spiritual, mental, and physical health. It is the Bible.

Some may doubt that this reference, so familiar to us, could possibly show how to have good mental and physical health, but there are people who have used it for this purpose for centuries with tremendous benefits. The principles discussed by the author have been proven to reduce the risk of many diseases, including cancer, diabetes, high cholesterol, obesity, and anxiety. These principles have been used to treat common diseases such as depression and hypertension.

Read the book you are holding and gain from the author's years of research in this subject. Learn how you can have true health by listening to the distant sound of wisdom.

Nick Walters, MD, DMT&H, FAAFP
Bangkok Adventist Hospital, Thailand

Preface

In this book current scientific information is presented in order to guide the reader toward a holistic approach to health. This is complemented by gems of wisdom coming from selected sages and prophets of the past. There is a surprisingly coherent pattern of advice coming from biblical writings in all the areas of human knowledge relevant to health issues today. A careful consideration of this information should increase the reader's appreciation of the authoritativeness of the Word of God. In fact, one of the main purposes of the book is to establish greater confidence in God's Word. If the advice is followed carefully, better health will be the reward. It is my fervent desire that readers will receive this reward too.

Good health is a commodity that is without price. When we lose our health, it is often difficult to retrieve it. If it is possible to regain health, the price tag can often be very high. As societies in emerging countries become a more effective part of the modern world community, the diseases that are readily communicated, such as trachoma, poliomyelitis, and measles, are becoming less damaging. The World Health Organization is active in reducing the disease burden in cooperation with partner nations. For example, it aims to eliminate trachoma by the year 2020, and it has made enormous progress in reducing the incidence of other communicable diseases. We are thankful that science has enabled us to make remarkable progress in controlling such damaging diseases.[1]

Now we are in a situation where non-communicable diseases are becoming more important. Already by 2001 it was estimated that around 46 percent of all deaths in the world were caused by chronic diseases, and by the year 2020 the figure is expected to be closer to 57 percent. The greatest burden of such diseases is being felt in developing countries. It is the faulty dietary habits and poor physical activity patterns that we are developing that accounts for the remarkable turnabout from interest in communicable diseases to non-communicable ones. Around half of the deaths through chronic diseases can be attributed to coronary heart disease, diabetes, and obesity. Diet-related diseases of interest also involve various forms of cancers. Other cancers are caused, not be faulty diet, but by tobacco use, accounting for 22 percent of global cancer deaths. It has been estimated that during this century 1000 million people will die as a result of smoking.[2]

The good news is that we can prevent most of these diseases by the lifestyle that we adopt. The most frequently cited dietary causes of the preventable diseases identified above are excess consumption of energy rich foods of animal origin and foods that contain added fat, sugar, and salt. Overweight develops quickly on such a calorie rich and unbalanced diet. In addition to obesity, the other lifestyle factors that contribute to ill health are smoking, stress, excessive alcohol consumption, and lack of physical activity.

In any concept of health, physical, mental, social, and spiritual aspects are involved. On a fundamental level I agree with the World Health Organization that health involves physical, mental, and social well-being.[3] In a more recent proposal, the Executive Board of the Organization recommended that "spiritual well-being" be included in the above definition.[4] Indeed, in a later statement it was held that "spiritual well-being can be thought of as a component of mental health…."[5] This reflects the idea that we need to recognize "the uniqueness of each person and the need to respond to each individual's spiritual quest for meaning, purpose and belonging."[6] However, in making these affirmative statements regarding the United Nations and their inclusion of spirituality as a component of mental health,

readers must not imagine that the writer supports initiatives by this and other bodies (e.g., United Religions Initiative) to create a world religion.

In this book the initial emphasis is in identifying dietary factors that are responsible for hastening the appearance of non-communicable diseases. Other lifestyle factors that lead to poor health will be highlighted together with environmental hazards. By identifying the underlying principles leading to health, the reader will then be in a good position to make wise choices. Finally, I will indicate that physical health alone does not hold the key to vibrant health. The domains of emotional, social, and spiritual health all contribute to our sense of well-being and our ability to function well in our families and communities. These facts are well recognized by the scientific community.

This book is my endeavor to provide information that, if followed, will contribute to good health in all areas of your life and increase your enjoyment.

References

[1] World Health Organization, "Trachoma," http://1ref.us/8e (accessed February 10, 2015); World Health Organization, "Poliomyelitis," (2014), http://1ref.us/8f (accessed February 10, 2015).

[2] Cancer Research, UK "Tobacco, Smoking and Cancer: the Evidence," (2009), http://1ref.us/8g (accessed February 10, 2015); World Health Organization, *Diet, Nutrition and the Prevention of Chronic Disease*, Technical Report Series 916 (Geneva: World Health Organization, 2003), 4–6; World Health Organization, "Cancer," (2014), http://1ref.us/8h (accessed February 10, 2015).

[3] World Health Organization, *Chronicle of the World Health Organization* 1, no. 1–2 (1947): 29.

[4] M. H. Khazat, "Spirituality in the Definition of Health. The World Health Organization Point of View," (c.1998), http://1ref.us/8i (accessed February 10, 2015).

[5] H. Herrman, S. Saxena and R. Moodie, eds, *Promoting Mental Health: Concepts, Emerging* *Evidence, Practice* (Geneva, Switzerland: World Health Organization, 2005), 55.

[6] D. Yach, *Ethik in der Medizin* 10 (1998): S7–S13, http://1ref.us/8j (accessed February 10, 2015).

Acknowledgments

The inspiration for writing a book may follow a convoluted path. After having completed several books on healthful living, both for serious Christians and those without leanings toward it, I considered that perhaps I had no more to contribute to the public in this area of knowledge. However, suggestions from several sources, including Jan, my wife, indicated that a different approach to the subject matter may be beneficial. Then, with the rapid increase in non-communicable diseases, many of which are diet-related, and with the increase, among some Christian believers, of a casual attitude toward the principles outlined in the Word of God, it became evident that something powerful could perhaps be said in defense of the Scriptures, which would result in both spiritual and physical health benefits.

Hence, I acknowledge the leading of God's Spirit along a pathway that has taken some years to reach clarity. It is perhaps unsurprising that having reached this point of finality I cannot clearly trace all the lines of my developing conviction and inspiration—some dawned slowly and others came with suddenness. However, two events I clearly remember. On a flight from Manila to Bangkok, I was inspired to sketch the initial outline of the document, and at a meeting in the theology department at Hong Kong Baptist University, the title of the book was impressed indelibly on my mind.

I am especially indebted to Pastor Don E. Bain, retired medical and health director, South Pacific Division of Seventh-day Adventists, for reading the text critically and making valuable suggestions. Without these the document would be weaker and sometimes less accurate.

Introduction

Chapter 1

Pythagoras, the Puritans, and Beyond

Pythagoras is known by every school graduate. We mention him here, but not for the reasons that usually bring his name to our notice. He is best known for his mathematical skills and his contributions to astronomy and harmonics, not his philosophy of life. Born around 580 BC on the Greek island of Samos, in the Aegean Sea, he was widely studied in the science and philosophy of the East and traveled to the great centers of learning. His concepts about the nature of humanity form a linking contrast with that held by the Puritans. He believed that a divine element (soul) was associated with the human body and furthermore that corrupt souls could reappear in other living creatures—in other words, the soul had the ability to transmigrate. This meant that efforts were made to purify the soul through rituals so as to achieve a status similar to the gods. Understandably, such a concept concerning the nature of humanity impacted his attitude toward animals and his dietary choices. The precise nature of these ideas is disputed, but conservative opinion is that he and his followers felt a certain kinship with animals and that at least some adherents did not eat meat.

There are echoes of these ideas in Vedic Hinduism and Mahayana Buddhism and other ancient religions. For example, certain Chinese scholars and monks (in the present era) equated Buddhism with vegetarianism and the practice flourished for a number of centuries. Now, the ethical principles of non-violence in the religion recommend this practice, as is the case in Taoism too.[1]

Moving on from Pythagoras, eventually the Greeks developed the idea that an individual consisted of a body and soul. The body was considered evil, while the soul basically was good. These ideas led some either to neglect or to treat the physical body roughly in order to purify it.[2] These ideas, in turn, influenced Christian thought.

The Puritans by contrast were a group of Christians in England (that arose in the 1560s) in whose ranks there were those who thought otherwise. They aimed at change in the government and organization of the Church of England in order to complete the work of the Reformation. The emphasis was on alterations to the structure and liturgy after the pattern of the Reformed Presbyterian Church. The overall incentive was to promote doctrinal purity and holiness of life. Puritan theology did not represent a consistent stream of thought, but within their ranks was a group that held strong opinions about body and spirit making up the whole person or soul; there was no immortal soul in this group's theology. They were unable to establish from the Bible that God infused a soul into the body at creation. Rather they believed that when God breathed into the body (molded out of the dust) that Adam became a living soul—a functioning, whole or complete human being. The central point in their arguments was that humans were mortal. The end result of such reasoning placed a renewed emphasis on the interrelations among the physical, mental, and spiritual aspects of living.[3] A critical look at Scripture will confirm this position as the one it upholds (Job 14:1, 2, 21; Psalm 115:17; 1 Corinthians 15:51–55; 1 Timothy 6:15, 16).

It is to the idea of the whole individual held by the Puritans and others, which has echoes in the modern concept of health, that we now turn our attention.

Complete Human Beings

The creation view of humanity is that humans are living souls or individuals but do not possess souls (Genesis 2:7). This was the Puritans' commencing point in their quest to understand God's will for everyday living. The concept was far removed from the Greek notion that the body is a prison house from which escape must be sought. The practical consequence of such a doctrine about the completeness of the human body for the Puritans was an advanced attitude toward health practices. They held the Bible view that the human body is God's temple (1 Corinthians 6:19).

The Bible outlines a comprehensive concept of wholeness involving the physical, mental, social, and spiritual elements.

The Bible outlines a comprehensive concept of wholeness involving the physical, mental, social, and spiritual elements. The words used to convey some ideas about wholeness are a little unusual and have a variety of meanings we often do not associate with health. The words are: *shalom*—wholeness, well-being, and peace (Genesis 37:14; 43:28; 1 Samuel 25:6); *gadosh*—holy, complete, and whole (Leviticus 11:44, 45); *tahor*—clean, pure, and genuine (Leviticus 13:17–20; 14:9; 2 Kings 5:14).[4] If we read Psalm 103 carefully, all these aspects of wholeness are mentioned. We notice in this psalm that David praises God for His benefits in giving physical health and spiritual peace (verses 3, 10–13). He invites the servants of God on earth and in the heavens to acknowledge the Lord for His greatness and goodness toward humanity and for His marvelous works (in other words God's servants are observing and thinking). Such combined praise highlights the social and mental aspects of health (verses 19–22). The whole psalm is in reality a hymn of optimism and thankfulness.

Health then involves all aspects of human existence and is inextricably involved in the pursuit of holiness (1 Corinthians 10:31),[5] a concept understood by some of the Puritans and others. For example, the well-known Baptist minister Oswald Chambers said: "God has only one intended destiny for mankind—holiness. His only goal is to produce saints…. Never tolerate, because of sympathy for yourself or others, any practice that is not in keeping with a holy God…. Holiness is not simply what God gives me, but what God has given me that is being exhibited in my life."[6] To those who follow this line of reasoning, several outcomes may be observed, including moderation of eating habits in both the quantity consumed and in the items selected for consumption. The logical conclusion reached by some of the Puritans was that a diet close to the one recommended by the Creator in Eden could be followed with confidence because the One who was holy had given the instructions in the beginning.[7]

Highlight: *Health involves physical, mental, social, as well as spiritual aspects of human existence.*

Dietary Choices

The dietary habits found in different countries vary widely and have arisen through a complex interaction of economic, climatic, philosophical, and other factors. The so-called Golden Age in early human history was a time of peaceful coexistence between humans and other creatures; people were nonviolent and vegetarian (Genesis 1:29; 3:18, 19).[8] This pattern changed after the great flood (Genesis 9:3, 4) when food scarcity was experienced.

Moving down through time, the staple diet of various people groups often evolved around wild plants and grains that were first harvested and then selectively grown and stored. Finally, domestication took place when these plants were systematically cultivated in areas somewhat removed from their wild relatives. This process can be deduced from studying the archeological records along the lower Yangtze and the Euphrates. In the former location, wild rice was first domesticated and latter barley, wheat, and rye were used.[9] Some dietary habits persisting to this day were developed early in some parts of the world. For example, the famous Mediterranean diet was known during the Hellenic era (323–31 BC). The staple food was barley supplemented with goat's milk, cheese, olives, figs, other fruits and vegetables, and fish. A variety of flours were available for bread making—barley, rice, and wheat. The use of meat among the general population was not abundant.[10]

The early Christians in the century of Christ's death and somewhat beyond probably lived on a diet of grains, vegetables, and dairy products and whatever meat they could obtain, just as the poor of Christian Europe are believed to have lived.[11] We well remember that Christ fed the multitudes following Him with barley loaves and fish (John 6:9–11). He undoubtedly ate lamb/kid at the Passover (Mark 14:14–16), and it is recorded that He ate bread and fish just before His ascension (John 21:13).

Some early writers have the apostles James, Matthew, and Peter living as vegetarians.

Some early writers have the apostles James, Matthew, and Peter living as vegetarians. Certainly, Tertullian (AD 160–240) approved of such practices and upheld Daniel the prophet (Daniel 1:8, 16) as his role model.[12] Whatever the truth of the claims about the apostles, for some time Christians refused to eat meat derived from the "unclean" or carnivorous/scavenging animals mentioned particularly in the Mosaic dietary code.[13] This was presumably because they understood that the distinction recorded by Moses had been recognized well before the Exodus experience (Genesis 7:2). The clear emphasis was that herbivorous animals and seed-eating birds were the closest to the creation ideal, since they shed no blood in satisfying their nutritional needs. Hence, the people felt it was safest to restrict their diet to these animals if adequate plant-derived food was not available.

In early Christianity, well after the time of the apostles, it has been testified that in contrast to the pagans, who clamored for blood (even human blood), that Christians did not eat blood and ate simply. Tertullian affirmed that they do "not [have] even the blood of animals at their meals of simple and natural food."[14]

While the Bible presents a flexible attitude toward eating the meat of animals that do not live by killing and scavenging activities, it is very clear about consuming their blood. The fact that New Testament believers understood that no blood was to be consumed even when these creatures were utilized (Acts 15:29) indicates that they kept vivid in their minds the idea that the Creator is the source of life and is holy. The apostle Peter, writing to the Christian church, urged all to "be holy in all *your* conduct" (1 Peter 1:15). He quoted as this authority Leviticus 11, verses 44 and 45, which comes to us at the end of Moses' account on unclean food. Clearly, this great individual understood that our eating and drinking had something to do with our spiritual experience.

The scientific soundness of avoiding blood will be commented upon later. At the same time as this advice comes to us, the Bible is not silent on another aspect impacting the choice of safe food. In the famous Bible story when the Hebrews hankered for meat during their wilderness journey to the land of Canaan (Exodus 16:3–13), quails were provided in abundance, and we are told the people ate greedily. Many of them died on account of their actions (Numbers 11:31–34). We can only speculate about their illness and death. They may have been poisoned by *Salmonella,* bacteria present in the birds that subsequently multiplied in the carcasses, or their illness may have been due to a toxin in seeds the birds may have eaten. Seeds of henbane (*Hyoscyamus niger*) are eaten by quail and may cause scopolamine poisoning. This condition was known in the ancient world and can occur following consumption of quail meat that has come from birds eating henbane seeds.[15]

The apostle Paul spoke about making wise food choices for another reason too (1 Corinthians 8:1–13; 10:28). His advice is often misunderstood, but one significant point might be mentioned here. He was adamant that the feelings of others should be considered when we make food selections so that we do not weaken their spiritual experience. This is good advice and it is not always followed. Indeed, history records that many were persecuted by the church fathers on account of their dietary choices.[16]

Highlights:

1. *Since the passing of the Golden Age in Eden, humans have consumed a variable amount of meat in their diets.*

2. *The Bible recommends that we make wise food choices and gives some guidance along these lines.*

3. *The early Christians ate simply.*

Section I: Physical Health

In our quest for health, we might do well to reflect on some of the wise sayings coming from the past. As we do this together, it will become evident that some philosophies and individual thinkers have long been in the territory where science is now taking us.

First, I will commence with some quotes from authors of note and then give several references from the Bible. The emphasis in the quotes is on physical health in this section, but it will soon become evident that physical health does not stand in isolation from other aspects of health. The existence of concise statements was one of the main factors used in selecting quotes for the reader's consideration.

Memorable Quotes[17]

"The health of the people is really the foundation upon which all their happiness and all their powers as a state depend" (Benjamin Disraeli).

"Walking is man's best medicine" (Hippocrates).

"In general, the more food we eat in its natural state—the less it is refined, and the fewer additives it contains—the healthier it will be for us. Food can affect the mind, and deficiencies in certain elements in the body can promote mental depression"
(Ezra Taft Benson).

"A human can be healthy without killing animals for food. Therefore if he eats meat he participates in taking animal life merely for the sake of his appetite"
(Leo Nikolaevich Tolstoy).

"Nothing will benefit human health and increase chances for survival on earth as the evolution to a vegetarian diet"
(Albert Einstein).

"And God said, 'See, I have given you every green herb that yields seed which on the face of the earth, and every tree whose fruit yields seed; to you it shall be for food'"
(Genesis 1:29).

"If you will listen carefully to the voice of the LORD your God and do what is right in his sight, obeying his commands and keeping all his decrees, then I will not make you suffer any of the diseases I sent on the Egyptians; for I am the LORD who heals you"
(Exodus 15:26, NLT).

"When you sit down to eat with a ruler, consider carefully what is before you; and put a knife to your throat if you are a man given to appetite. Do not desire his delicacies, for they are deceptive food" (Proverbs 23:1–3).

Chapter 2

Prospering and in Good Health

Health interests people irrespective of the country they live in. This interest is reflected both in the popular and scientific press. The place of nutrition in good health is well established. Nutrition involves the intake of nutrients, their digestion, absorption, subsequent breakdown and, finally, the elimination of waste products. Failure in any of these areas will have an impact on health.

The basic nutrients needed by the body are carbohydrates, proteins, fats, vitamins, minerals, and water. All these nutrients must be in the correct amount, otherwise optimal health will not be experienced. The main role of carbohydrates is to provide energy. They come in a wide variety of foods such as rice, noodles, potatoes, maize, cassava, and many others. They are broken down by the enzymes present in the body to provide glucose, and this allows the energy generating processes to function well. Complex carbohydrates (starches and cell wall materials derived from plants) are more difficult to break down than simple carbohydrates such as sugars. This means that they release energy more slowly. The breakdown products of carbohydrates function as carbon-containing building block molecules that are essential for the construction of new cells.[18] In making these new cells, nitrogen-containing building block molecules are also required.

Nitrogen is provided principally by proteins (mainly contained in meat, eggs, milk, legumes, and nuts). Proteins are composed of amino acids. It is important to note that nine of these cannot be manufactured in the human body in sufficient quantity to maintain health and must be consumed in the food we eat. Proteins are not our main source of energy. Their role is in the construction and repair of cells, and in addition, they provide components of the working machinery in the cells. Excess protein has been associated with the formation of kidney stones, early kidney failure, cardiac function impairment, increased cancer risk, and osteoporosis. High protein foods that have a high fat content are associated with obesity, greater incidence of cardiovascular disease, and decreased lifespan. The best advice is to prefer a high carbohydrate, low protein diet. In practice this means using high quality protein (15–20 percent of total calorie intake) together with good quality complex carbohydrates. This will deliver better cardiac health and promote longer life.[19]

Fats are essential nutrients too. They are found in plant and animal foods and are composed of fatty acids and glycerol. These components are required for the integrity of the cell membranes (or envelope). If the membranes are not constructed well and do not remain intact, an individual will not continue to remain healthy. Now, membranes are involved in the production and storage of energy.

Two essential fatty acids cannot be made in the body. These are linoleic and linolenic acids. They are found in both animal and plant sources. For those preferring a vegetarian lifestyle, adequate quantities can be found in vegetables, nuts, grains, and fruits.[20] While speaking about fats, we need to understand the difference between saturated and unsaturated/polyunsaturated fats. The fats that are saturated are typically solid at room temperature (i.e., 25°C.) whereas the unsaturated fats are typically soft or liquid at this temperature. Over-consumption of fats, and particularly some types of saturated fats, is of worldwide concern, for it leads to diseases of the heart and other organs. On the other hand, not all products derived from polyunsaturated fats are beneficial (i.e., trans fats). Liquid oils that have been made into solid

fat by the process of bubbling hydrogen through oil (hydrogenation) contain trans fats (commonly found in fast foods and bakery products). These fats aid in the elevation of cholesterol levels.[21]

Vitamins and minerals are nutrients required by the body in small amounts. The vitamins are either fat soluble (A, D, E, K) or water soluble (B complex and C). Excessive intake of fat soluble vitamins can cause toxicity, which will injure us. Vitamins do not act as a source of energy but participate in essential cell functions, and their absence will lead to a number of diseases. Minerals are required in either moderate or in trace amounts. These also assist in keeping the machinery of the cell working properly. Their absence or sometimes excess will cause various health problems to develop.[22]

Highlight: *Carbohydrates, proteins, fats, vitamins, and minerals when balanced and taken in moderation promote health.*

Besides all these nutrients, water is required for the transport of nutrients and wastes and is essential to the general functioning of the cell. The role of water in the regulation of body temperature is critical.[23]

In the following section, I examine how a balance in nutrient intake may be maintained.

Animal and Plant-Based Diets

The human race has used both plants and animals for food since antiquity. The vegetarian way of life was the one originally designed for the benefit of humanity as explained in the book of Genesis. Following the creation of the human race, God wisely indicated how the delicate and complex organism might be cared for. He indicated that fruits and vegetables were specifically designed to keep the body in peak condition (Genesis 1:29). In fact, it was some time after the entrance of sin and destruction of a sizable proportion of earth's evil inhabitants that God gave instructions indicating meat might be used. It was set aside for the use of humans in the altered circumstances, which was marked by a drastic reduction in the availability of food resources (Genesis 8:13–17; 9:3). Not surprisingly, in the New Earth, which God will create after the reign of sin has been terminated, meat eating will disappear. And this will apply to both animals and humans. The Bible is very clear that carnivorous animals will have a spectacular makeover (Isaiah 65:17, 25).

Vegetarianism is something that has been promoted by various groups of people for thousands of years. However, in recent years the scientific community has come to realize that the vegetarian lifestyle has much to recommend it. Studies commenced almost fifty years ago have shown rather convincingly that a plant-based diet leads to a healthier and longer life than one based on meat.[24] The World Health Organization has predicted that by the year 2020 two-thirds of the global incidence of disease will be attributable to chronic non-communicable diseases. Most of these diseases will be caused by over nutrition through overeating animal products and increased consumption of refined foods and fats. All this is happening within an environment that does not encourage us to have sufficient exercise.[25]

The World Health Organization has predicted that by the year 2020 two-thirds of the global incidence of disease will be attributable to chronic non-communicable diseases.

Readers of this book may not wish to follow the example of various thought leaders and scientists of note in adopting a non-meat or minimal meat diet. They may prefer to adopt a flexible diet with abundant choice of fruits and vegetables supplemented by meat either occasionally or regularly. However, in all life's choices it is best to be informed about the adequacy of a vegetarian diet so that wise decisions can be made. The adequacy of this diet has been answered in relation to a number of points.

Protein Adequacy

Certain essential amino acids must be taken into the body because it cannot manufacture them itself. Good health is dependent on the regular supply of nine essential amino acids in the diet. These amino acids are generally close to balance in animal products and are termed high-quality proteins. A few plant proteins are in this league too (soy, quinoa, and amaranth). Studies have shown that growth of children on a lacto-ovo-vegetarian diet (dairy products and eggs included) can hardly be distinguished from those on a meat diet.[26] An interesting finding is that plant-based diets are able to supply the protein needs of serious athletes so that their performance is indistinguishable from their meat-eating counterparts.[27]

In a plant-based diet, intake of a variety of proteins from different sources each day will provide balanced nutrition. This means, in practice, that cereals and legumes in combination will provide adequate proteins. Soy protein supplies all the essential amino acids, giving it first priority on the menu as the king among several plant protein choices.[28] The protein needs of vegetarians may be higher than the Recommended Dietary Allowance if the source of protein comes from limited plant sources. However, when mixed plant sources are used, the protein requirements do not differ from those shown by meat eaters.[29] In contrast to plant proteins, animal proteins may be rich in sulfur-based amino acids, and these increase the risk of osteoporosis. Bone loss from vegetarians is less than from non-vegetarians, which is also related partly to the consumption of soy products.[30] Neglected sources of proteins with some individuals and in selected cultures are species of edible mushroom. They contain most of the essential amino acids and minerals, B vitamins, and folic acid.[31] In fact, one fungal meat substitute has been perfected that rivals eggs in its amino acid composition.[32] We should not confuse edible mushrooms with poisonous mushrooms or microscopic fungi that are capable of producing toxins in numerous foods. If we do this, we may end up condemning all fungi, which is unreasonable and beyond the evidence.

In the extensive European study involving 22,000 individuals with various dietary habits, it was found that meat eaters had the highest body mass index (BMI) with vegans the lowest. Those who practiced a vegetarian lifestyle and fish eaters showed intermediate BMIs. This is good news for those attempting to control obesity. The good news does not stop there but extends to a reduced incidence of cardiovascular disease, type 2 diabetes, and kidney disease in those using plant protein.[33] However, BMI is not the single indicator of risk. Not all overweight or obese people contract metabolic diseases such as diabetes.[34]

Essential Fatty Acids

The two essential fatty acids required by humans are linoleic and linolenic. These cannot be synthesized in the human body, but are required for a variety of vital functions. There is some possibility that vegetarians and vegans may be disadvantaged, particularly among pregnant and lactating women. Adequate plant sources of both fatty acids exist (linoleic—corn, safflower, sunflower, and peanut oils, almonds, etc.; linolenic—seed oils such as soybean and canola). This means that judicious choices need to be made or the diet needs to be supplemented with oily fish, eggs, milk, sea vegetables, or seed oils.[35]

Minerals

Various issues have been raised. First, the calcium status of vegetarians has been questioned. The fact is that bone mineral density may be either higher or lower in vegetarians than meat eaters. Where soy products are consumed regularly and where high protein, salt rich diets are avoided, then calcium intake tends to be adequate. This is especially true if the diet change is combined with exercise and alcohol and smoking are avoided.[36] Vegans need to pay special attention to their calcium intake otherwise their risk of bone fracture will increase.[37]

The question of iron deficiency is also worth discussing because it is often thought that vegetarians and vegans are more likely to experience problems acquiring iron. Now iron deficiency often is associated with anemia. When individuals are anemic, they lack energy and are listless and are susceptible to infection by disease organisms. Animal products contain heme and non-heme iron. Plants on the other hand contain non-heme iron, and it is not absorbed as readily as heme iron found in meats (heme is a complex, red organic pigment containing iron and other atoms to which oxygen binds). However, vitamins A and C, and a range of organic acids found in plants, aid in the absorption of non-heme iron by the body. All this means that with a mixed diet of grains, legumes and nuts, fruits, and vegetables, there is no difficulty in meeting the iron needs of the body. Vegetarians (irrespective of their intake of milk products and eggs) are well able to meet their iron requirements. However, some difficulties may be experienced with children on a restricted macrobiotic diet (mainly whole grains and vegetables based on the Ayurvedic tradition) and by rice eaters who extensively use common Green Revolution varieties.[38]

Insufficient supplies of other minerals do not occur commonly in the West.[39] However, it has been estimated that about a third of the world's population may suffer from zinc deficiency. This mineral is required in trace amounts for many essential body functions. The requirement for the mineral is well catered for in vegetarians by sun-dried tomatoes, soy products, and other legumes, nuts, whole grain cereals, and certain seeds (pumpkin, sunflower, and sesame). It is found in lean meats, cheese, milk, and eggs. The risk of encountering zinc deficiency appears to be no greater among vegetarians and non-vegetarians in Western societies. In some other societies, food-processing techniques may not be available to reduce the amount of phytic acid from plant sources, which is inhibitory to zinc absorption.[40]

There is perhaps one other mineral that merits a brief mention and that is iodine. With the common availability of iodized salt in many countries, this should not be a problem there—this is not to forget that around 700 million people suffer from brain damage and retardation though through lack of adequate supplies of the mineral. For those who avoid iodized salt, then either sea vegetables or other good sources of the mineral such as soybeans, sweet potatoes, and cruciferous vegetables are recommended.[41]

Vitamins

People living in the fast lane often tend to eat junk food, which has a high fat and salt content and excess simple sugars. Simple sugars and refined foods (e.g., white sugar and flour) come stripped of their vitamins and minerals. The vitamins in the spotlight are A, B_{12}, and folic acid. These are present in meat or have a better bioavailability in meat than in plants. Low vitamin B_{12} levels have been measured in vegetarians and vegans in a number of studies. It is, in fact, a worldwide problem.[42] This vitamin is found in animal-based foods (red meats, poultry, dairy and derived products, fish, and fermented fish sauce). Lacto-ovo-vegetarians may obtain adequate supplies from eggs, cheese, milk, and yogurt, but vegans are at particular risk.

The adequacy of non-animal sources of B_{12} for humans is contested in some circles.

The adequacy of non-animal sources of B_{12} for humans is contested in some circles (readers must remember that there are active and inactive forms of B_{12}). Inactive forms are no use, so false claims can be made. Adequate quantities of the active form appear to have been found in some seaweeds (green and purple laver) and shiitake mushrooms. Other sources are found in tempe, kimchi, and fermented black tea. On the basis of the evidence available, in many parts of the world adequate source of the vitamin are available consistently only from fortified plant sources.[43]

Vitamin B_{12} is required to prevent anemia and irreversible nervous system damage in the fetus as well as neurological disorders in the aging. It is no small matter to think of the legacy one can give in ensuring adequate supplies of this vitamin are supplied to infants. The Vegan Society recognizes this. For those who cannot eat animal, fortified soy milk, or other products, they should supplement their intake through the use of tablets or by using fortified foods. The need for supplementation is higher in some countries than others, which is a reflection of the dietary habits adopted and the amount of meat consumed. In developed countries, individuals over fifty years of age (irrespective of their food preferences) often require supplementation in order to avoid deficiency.[44]

The question of vitamin B_{12} deficiency in plants has caused some to question the adequacy of the diet provided by God to the newly created couple in Eden. One highly significant fact that we must bear in mind in answering this question is that we are no longer in Eden, and many changes have come upon the human race and the earth as a result of the curses that have been experienced as a result of sin (Genesis 3:16, 17; 4:12; cf. 9:3, 4). That having been said, I have no completely adequate answer as to how supplies of this vitamin were provided originally, as no plant or animal synthesizes a bioavailable form of the vitamin (classically it is regarded as a bacterial product). However, it has been noted in some disease states that the blood levels of this vitamin and folic acid are elevated due to excessive growth of bacteria in portion of the small intestine usually supporting poor bacterial growth on account of the high acidity of that environment.[45] This suggests that the delicate balance of microbes in the intestines may have changed after the fall, accounting for difficulties now seen in humans.

Turning now to other vitamins, animal products contain preformed vitamin A whereas plants contain the starting molecule (beta-carotene) that is required for its synthesis. Plants high in beta-carotene are the bright colored orange fruits and vegetables (carrots, pumpkins, tomatoes, mango, papaya, apricot, etc.) and dark green ones (spinach, broccoli, cabbage, lettuce, etc.). This vitamin is not usually deficient in diets of people in Western countries, but this is not true of many Asian communities.[46]

Folic acid deficiencies may lead to anemia and to birth defects (neural tube). A range of fruits, vegetables, and meat supply folate. Supplementation of grain products is carried out in some countries to overcome deficiency problems developing.[47] In some Asian countries, multivitamins are handed out to pregnant women in an attempt to reduce the risk of premature birth, to develop the nerve cells, and to strengthen the immune system.[48] This appears to be a wise practice.

Highlight: A plant-based diet provides adequate nutrition. Special attention needs to be given to the intake of several vitamins.

Regardless of our motivation, there are several additional advantages that we might expect

through adopting a plant-based diet. These are as follows: fat intake, fiber intake, phytochemicals, and foodborne disease.

Fat Intake

The difference in fat intake between vegetarians and meat eaters is usually substantial. Not only do vegetarians consume less fat, but it contains less saturated fat and cholesterol. It is no secret that fat intake and poor health are closely related, for dietary fat is efficiently converted to body fat, and this increases disease risk. Calories acquired through fat intake should make up less than 30 percent. Furthermore, the calories contributed to by saturated fat should be less than 10 percent.[49]

Fish have a special place in many cultures. The scientific information tells us that this food item contains special beneficial fatty acids (omega-3). Intake of omega-3 fatty acids was first associated with lowered risk of heart attacks among Eskimos. They also have beneficial effects in lowering chronic inflammatory diseases and mortality due to cancer. Significantly they promote eye and brain development.

As fish sources dwindle and their price increases, it is good to know that there are plant sources of omega-3 fatty acids. These are found in nuts, seeds, and beans (flaxseed, walnuts, and canola oil are particularly high in these fatty acids; soybeans and tofu contain moderate amounts). This means that the beneficial effects of these oils may be enjoyed without having to worry about possible heavy metal and other contaminants and pathogens present in some fish today.[50] To illustrate, some species of fish contain significant quantities of methylmercury, polychlorinated biphenyls, dioxins, and other damaging chemicals. This is particularly the case amongst predatory fish and mammals where the substances present in the environment are magnified through the feeding behavior of the fish (biomagnifications occurs).[51] It is of interest to note that the Dietary Guidelines for Americans Advisory Committee believes the risks associated with the intake of pollutants through eating two servings per week as recommended outweigh the benefits. Hence, they advise a lower weekly intake (340g) and restriction in the use of large, predatory fish.[52]

Fiber Intake

Fruits and vegetables are higher in fiber content (i.e., plant carbohydrates that essentially are indigestible). The advantage of fiber is that digestive complaints are reduced such as constipation and diverticular disease (protrusions of the inner lining of the intestines). The rate of glucose absorption also is slowed, and thus fiber intake is beneficial for diabetics as well as to non-diabetics. The added bonus is that the risk of developing colorectal cancer and heart disease is lowered. Transit times of material through the digestive tract are shortened by the presence of insoluble fiber that adds bulk to the diet, accounting for the positive effect on colorectal cancer incidence. The effect of fiber on heart disease reduction is through the ability of soluble fiber to lower serum cholesterol (LDL) levels. Oat bran and psyllium are particularly high in soluble fiber.[53]

Phytochemicals

Positive health outcomes are associated with vegetarianism through the intake of a range of plant chemicals. The prospects are too good to ignore, but more information is needed before spectacular claims are made. In the meantime, health conscious individuals should eat fruits and vegetables as often as possible. One protective effect of soy products that we have noted already is that they minimize bone calcium loss. They also are thought to reduce the incidence of certain cancers and in individuals with high cholesterol levels the plant sterols that soy products contain can lower these levels.[54]

There is also evidence that some plant-based chemicals are beneficial in clearing the body of reactive oxygen and nitrogen entities produced in it. The former are produced in larger quantities when the body utilizes oxygen at high rates, such as during strenuous exercise or work, or in certain disease states and when selected environmental pollutants are abundant. This means, in practical terms, that stressed and non-stressed people should consider eating a balanced diet with plenty of fruits and vegetables added. However, there is no clinical evidence to confirm that vitamin and antioxidant supplementation is beneficial in reducing heart-associated diseases. The good news is that when we restrict the intake of calories into the body we also reduce free radical production, and when we undertake regular exercise, we strengthen our protection against damaging oxidants.[55] These byproducts of metabolism may destroy cell components and interfere with cell function. Drinking antioxidant rich products (black grape, raspberry, red currant) after exercise reduces the level of damage.[56]

Foodborne Disease

The association between foodborne disease and meat eating is strong. The most spectacular outbreaks of disease and deaths usually have been associated with foods that are not of plant origin. Having said this, it is important to notice that disease outbreaks are being increasingly associated with plant-based products on account of the ways they are produced, processed, and marketed. This concern is real, but limited.[57]

Highlights:

1. *A plant-based diet provides less fat and a healthier type of fat than meats and fewer diseases are associated with plant foods.*

2. *Special protective substances are found in plants against disease.*

Our nutritional needs at birth are different from those in adolescence and old age. I do not need to dwell on this point too much, but I will mention several points relevant to dietary habits. Calcium loss from bones on aging is particularly a problem in Western societies. This is a consequence of kidney dysfunction. If they do not remove sufficient phosphorus from the blood or turn vitamin D into the active form, then calcium is lost from the bones. Caffeine consumption increases the loss of calcium, and soy and other bean products and leafy vegetables lower the risk of bone calcium loss and fracture.

In some studies, vegetarians have been shown to have an advantage over meat eaters as far as bone mineral mass loss is concerned, but the picture is complex and depends on the dietary patterns. Suffice it to say that calcium balance is a greater problem in aging people and supplementation may be required when calcium intakes are low. The other nutrients requiring comment are vitamins B_{12} and D. Absorption of this particular B vitamin declines with age so that supplementation is recommended. Vitamin D synthesis declines markedly with age, requiring increased sun exposure (three to six times longer in dark skinned people than fair skinned) or intake of fortified foods. Low dose mineral supplements for zinc deficiency in older persons are also recommended.[58] Caution needs to be exercised by pregnant vegan and vegetarian mothers to enable an adequate intake of all these nutrients in addition to iron and magnesium.[59]

Highlights:

1. *Calcium loss from bones is less in vegetarians than meat eaters.*

2. *Vegetarians need to be nutritionally intelligent about vitamin intake particularly during pregnancy and old age.*

In the following section, I will address some understandings of various groups of people found in their writings in order to indicate that not all useful information arose in the present scientific age.

Some Beneficial Practices

Some groups of people choose a diet based on plants because this represents the ways of their traditional culture. Others adopt this lifestyle on account of religious beliefs or due to the sanctity that is attributed to all life forms or, more recently, on account of concerns about the sustainability of the planet using present methods of producing food (Genesis 1:29; Isaiah 65:17, 25).[60]

The broad principles understood by indigenous peoples recorded in their writings or handed down as practical knowledge are capable of preventing some illnesses. We do not claim that this should be the sole source of modern knowledge, but there is still much to learn from long established practices by indigenous people. For example, modern science agrees with the broad sweep of the advice found in the ancient Jewish writings, as illustrated in the best seller "None of These Diseases."[61] In contrast to some modern writers, I believe that a workable interface already exists between science and philosophy; there is a unity of knowledge. This means there is no need to anxiously wait for inspired hope to emerge in the future.[62]

Modern science agrees with the broad sweep of the advice found in the ancient Jewish writings.

I will examine some examples to illustrate this point of view. The biblical account of the story about origins suggests that a personal, loving God made humans and instructed them to use fruit and seed bearing cereals and herbs (Genesis 1:29). In other words, the Creator left instructions on diet much as a car maker provides a service manual. These plant-based foods that He gave the human race would have come fresh from the field. If this account is sound, then we might expect modern scientific data to give credibility to the idea that increasing these components in the diet contributes to good health. It is fascinating to note that modern science gives broad support to the practice of eating largely of fruits and vegetables in a natural state as a way to maximize the experience of good health.

Refined or highly processed food came to be used relatively late by the human race. If we observe the practices prevailing in some rural areas of Asia and the Pacific as examples, we still notice that the indigenous people use relatively few refined products. Refined products present us with a number of unwelcome problems as illustrated in a study comparing the health of selected groups of people in rural and semi-rural China with the health of other people who had chosen to eat according to 'modern' ways. The diseases formerly associated with affluence, which are cancer, diabetes, and coronary heart disease, are found commonly in eaters of modern foods or in those communities where traditional foods and lifestyles are changing rapidly.[63] Then, too, the increased incidence of asthma and allergies identified in developed countries has been linked provisionally to the intake of fast foods. The adoption of a Mediterranean diet or similar is beneficial in avoiding or minimizing these conditions.[64]

Various preservation techniques were developed by ancient peoples as knowledge increased and food security became an issue. Butter and cheese were early items discovered by the human race. Seeds and fruits were dried for preservation and fermentation was known from early times.

Historians record other methods of preservation practiced by past generations.[65] The use of salted food was valued early as a trading item and part of its attraction was as a preservative. As we look at these methods of preservation—drying, salting, and fermentation—we notice that they have not been without their special problems. For example, high salt in the diet has been associated with higher levels of stroke and cardiovascular disease. Calcium excretion in urine is increased through its use, thus aggravating the tendency toward brittle bones (osteoporosis). Increased salt intake is closely related to increased incidences of hypertension and stroke. In fact, some individuals with elevated blood pressure can improve their health status simply by reducing salt intake.[66]

Highlight: Many indigenous people and those holding to some ancient religious traditions based on the concept of a creator God use a largely plant-based diet containing few refined and processed products and are healthier as a result.

In some Western countries, around half of the calories taken in come from refined foods that are deficient in fiber, vitamins, and minerals. An associated issue is over consumption. This means that in such societies the leading causes of death are associated with a faulty diet.[67] Unfortunately, refined foods and sugar-laced drinks are two of the practices almost immediately taken on by developing countries in our trade-liberated world. This problem is now seen emerging in all societies taking on westernized ways. Whatever eating styles we choose, extremes will injure the chances of good health. Moderation in eating habits is called for at all times.[68] Obesity is really a disorder of energy balance. If the intake of energy exceeds the amount needed by the body, then obesity results. It is true that there are genetic factors that influence weight control, but the intake of food is highly significant.[69]

What we need is nutritional intelligence. Perhaps a good statement applicable to westernized countries and those attracted to its ways is the one given by an Eastern wise man from antiquity. It was King Solomon who said, "A curse shall not come upon any one without a cause" (Proverbs 26:2, Septuagint). This statement resonates with a well-known line from Buddhist culture that says, "Every human being is the author of his own health or disease."[70] In the Western world and certain sections of the Eastern world, there is a wealth of scientific information available urging us to make sensible nutritional choices. We should have little excuse in missing the information designed to prevent us from falling victim to nutritional deficiencies and related problems. In non-westernized areas of the world, traditional lifestyles often have much to recommend them, especially where they are based largely on plant products with low intake of meat.

Highlights:
1. *Refined foods are usually deficient in fiber, vitamins, and minerals.*
2. *Moderation in food intake will promote a healthier and longer life.*

I sound a note of advice here. We should not assume that either indigenous cultures or scientists have captured all the wisdom that is available. Nutritional deficiencies are found commonly among plants as well as animals. This means that we should be very careful about claims concerning the total adequacy of a vegetable based diet without supplementation in all parts of the world or extravagant claims about a particular food item. We might equally be careful about the adequacy of some traditional storage methods. Selected stored products contribute to shortened lifespans due to intake of toxic materials generated in them that exert long-term effects on health. This has been observed particularly in the tropics where stored

food items allow microbes to grow on account of the moist environment. The toxins produced may be very powerful and may predispose to disease, including cancer.[71]

> *We should be very careful about claims concerning the total adequacy of a vegetable based diet without supplementation in all parts of the world.*

Balanced Eating

There are members in every society who have too little to eat, and there are some countries where few have an adequate supply of food. However, as economies strengthen, access to abundant, attractive food is increasing. This is not a problem that has suddenly come upon the human race. In ancient civilizations the aristocratic and privileged classes were faced with the issue of overeating and were exposed to the health problems that followed. The wise man Solomon, who had experience in some Eastern cultures in ancient times, had this to say: "When you sit down with a ruler, consider carefully what *is* before you; and put a knife to your throat if you *are* a man given to appetite. Do not desire his delicacies, for they *are* deceptive food" (Proverbs 23:1–3). His advice was not to overeat, something that is clearly understood in Buddhist, Islamic, and some Christian teachings (Proverbs 23:1–3; 25:27).[72] This wisdom is something that many in the Western world, and to an increasing extent in other societies, could profitably note. It is a well-recorded fact that food portion sizes have increased together with fast foods. This trend was observed commencing particularly in the United States.[73] Other westernized countries, or those attracted to Western style fast foods, are also facing an epidemic of obesity. Indeed, it is noted that China and India now vie for the title of the diabetes capital of the world. The food choices we make carry their own health time bomb.[74]

How deceptive some foods are is now being discovered. It is hardly possible to call fast foods fine foods, but the principle stated for fine foods applies equally well to fast foods that are eaten in increasing abundance. These foods tend to be sweet and/or fatty and salty. This represents the worst possible combination for maintaining health.[75] Just a few fatty meals can start the downward spiral, as the hormone system appears to adjust itself to crave more fat. Overdosing on sugary foods has an addictive-like effect and has other repercussions as well.[76]

Simple sugars, if taken in abundance, are not good for health whether they are natural products or extracts from plants such as cane sugar. For example, honey is composed primarily of simple sugars (fructose and glucose) and will do its part in promoting various diseases, such as diabetes and tooth decay. The same might be said of soft drinks and some processed fruit juices that contain added sugar. Such decay results when the bacteria found in our mouths use sugars in food to produce organic acids. These acids simply decalcify the enamel, and this hastens cavity formation.[77] We will look at diabetes in another chapter. The simple truth is that the more refined the food the quicker the food is digested and the sooner blood glucose will rise. If we swamp the body with simple sugars, we are well on the road to ill health.[78]

Proteins are needed by the body. High protein diets commonly advocated by Atkins and others exert many adverse consequences; proteins are best taken in moderation.[79] Eating high protein, high fat diets does not have the support of a majority of nutritionists. Individuals with mild kidney insufficiency are particularly at risk of further damaging these organs through high protein intake.[80] There is an additional suggestion that fertility may be lowered by high protein diets.[81] A simple way in which to think about nutrition is to consider a building construction site. Building materials are required in various proportions—steel, wood, concrete, etc. If too much steel is supplied to a building site, it has to be removed with inconvenience and expense. The body is no different. The cells of the body are made up of various structural elements. If too much of a particular nutrient is supplied to the body, adverse consequences will be experienced, as some organs will have to work harder to remove or store it somewhere. And crowding the body with unwanted materials, such as fat, will bring its own penalty.

If too much of a particular nutrient is supplied to the body, adverse consequences will be experienced.

Highlights:

1. *Sweet, fatty, and salty foods are injurious to health.*

2. *High protein and high fat diets lead to poor health.*

Balanced eating together with moderate and regular exercise helps to keep us in good health and at the same time allows us to maintain our personal enjoyment. In fact, our enjoyment of food is heightened by recognizing that there is a spiritual dimension to our lives. An expression of this thought by one well-known writer is as follows: "A person can do nothing better than to eat and drink and find satisfaction in their own toil. This too, I see, is from the hand of God, for without him, who can eat or find enjoyment?" (Ecclesiastes 2:24, 25, NIV).

Beyond Nutrition?

Before I leave this chapter, one principle uncovered by modern science must be highlighted. Certain genetic abnormalities and mutations can mean that loss of vigor and vitality will be a person's lot in life irrespective of their dietary habits. Such individuals have done nothing to deserve their poor health. Examples of diseases due to genetic disorders are Crohn's disease, cystic fibrosis, Down syndrome, celiac disease, and others.[82] Even here, however, nutrition cannot be neglected. Cystic fibrosis provides an example where careful attention to nutrition, monitoring health, and controlling weight gain are essential to retaining some quality of life.[83] The debilitating effects of celiac disease can be avoided by carefully choosing cereal protein sources.[84]

In instances where genetic predisposition plays a role in the incidence of disease,[85] there may be several ways in which the risks of developing the disease can be minimized. We might illustrate this by reference to benign tumor detection in the large intestine and removal through colonoscopy as a measure to prevent the ultimate development of bowel cancer. Then in Western countries, and to an increasing extent elsewhere, screening for selected cancers is benefiting many with the gift of longer life. At the same time as these minimization strategies are being adopted, particularly with cancer-related illnesses, there are nutritional strategies that can impact the outcome positively too. I will highlight this in other chapters.

Guiding Principles and Practical Suggestions

1. Some of the broad principles understood by indigenous peoples recorded in their writings or handed down as practical knowledge are capable of preventing some illnesses. Traditional diets that have much to recommend them are those that include plenty of fruits and vegetables and contain little meat. Natural foods when taken from a variety of sources are best suited to supply our nutritional needs.

2. A vegetarian diet adequately provides for human nutritional needs and is healthier than an animal-based diet. A plant-based diet provides more fiber, less fat and reduced exposure to foodborne diseases than an animal-based diet. It also provides helpful phytochemicals. Proteins supplied by plants are able to supply all our needs; they are less commonly associated with the so-called diseases of affluence.

3. Staple carbohydrates retain the greatest quantities of fiber, essential nutrients, and key vitamins when they are minimally processed. This means that unpolished rice is more nutritious than polished or white rice. Minimally processed wheat and maize will deliver a better health outcome than food items based on finely ground and highly processed flour.

4. Fresh, brightly colored and green fruits and vegetables provide abundant sources of vitamins A and C.

5. Foods laden with fats, simple sugars, and salt contribute to ill health when eaten continually.

6. Extremes in eating will injure the chances of good health. Moderation in eating habits is called for at all times. Overeating and the abundant use of refined, custom-made food are deleterious to maintaining good health.

7. Overconsumption of protein is deleterious to health. The rules that apply to the construction of cells inform us that the unbalancing of carbohydrates to nitrogen containing nutrients overburden the liver and kidneys. A

good rule is that proteins should not exceed 10–20 percent of calories and should be low in fat. Carbohydrates used should be of the complex type.[86]

8. Some vitamin and mineral supplements may be required as we age or if we choose to be strict vegetarians. The latter group particularly needs to pay attention to vitamin B_{12} supplies. Zinc deficiency may develop in older persons who wish to be vegetarians. This mineral may be supplied by eating beans, nuts, wholegrain cereals, wheat germ, and tofu.

9. Disease risk minimization can be accomplished for some conditions through careful attention to diet, but others are unaffected.

Chapter 3

Preserving Stability

The Spanish explorer Juan Ponce de Leon made a serious attempt in 1513 to discover the place called the Fountain of Youth. Needless to say he never succeeded, and he died at the relatively young age of sixty-one years.[87] The modern explorer may more realistically find the secret of long life at the supermarket or village food market when armed with the correct information.

Analysis of the risk factors associated with good health has indicated that both food and regular exercise have significant impacts on life expectancy. In fact, regular exercise can be more important than dietary factors. Life expectancy is also influenced by adequate sleep, abstaining from tobacco, limiting alcohol intake, maintaining body weight close to the recommended, not snacking, and eating a regular breakfast. Individuals who are aware of these associations and make the appropriate lifestyle choices are likely to live seven or more years longer.[88] There are some lifestyle groups that enjoy additional years of life because they avoid harmful substances such as tobacco and alcohol and their philosophy embraces a healthy lifestyle including vegetarianism as the dietary ideal.

One extensive study conducted over eight years in California involving 25,000 individuals (Seventh-day Adventists), who choose a vegetarian lifestyle (adhering to the biblical model), showed a striking record of longer and healthier lives. The incidence of coronary heart disease, stroke, cancer, and diabetes was close to half that of other Californians. Follow-up studies among a mixed group of around 73,000 in the same location showed lower levels of heart, renal, and endocrine diseases among vegetarians. In other studies, the advantages of a vegetarian lifestyle have been shown to be independent of the country in which the study was conducted. The higher the amounts of red meat, fatty foods, eggs, and coffee consumed by the survey group, the greater their risk of early death. The take-home message is that those who keep to their recommended weight range, exercise, and eat a diet high in fruits and vegetables, and essentially avoid meat, can expect to live longer. The sooner that such a lifestyle is adopted the better. In fact, it has been established recently that the structural integrity of chromosomes is maintained by such practices, which accounts for the longer life experienced.[89]

The higher the amounts of red meat, fatty foods, eggs, and coffee consumed...the greater their risk of early death.

Highlight: *A vegetarian lifestyle can give up to seven or more years of enjoyable life. Mediterranean and Asian diets are also known for their life-extending benefits.*

The people surveyed evidently were living in harmony with their environment and enjoyed the results of doing so. This is not a new thought. The Greek philosopher Pythagoras who lived 500 years before the present era was devoted to the idea of maintaining stability or living in a harmonious state with nature as a virtue.[90] He also was dedicated to the vegetarian ideal.[91] A similar idea is supported by some Buddhist communities[92] and others. The concept of maintaining stability also is encompassed broadly in the modern idea of homeostasis. This concept recognizes that in the natural biological world stable conditions are maintained by inbuilt processes, such as seen in an animal body or a living cell. This means that an organism can operate in a broad range of environmental conditions without losing control. I will show how dietary choices can either assist in maintaining balance or in throwing the body into an unbalanced state. However, first I will look at some dietary choices available.

Dietary Choices

There are several diet types that we might adopt in our modern, developed world. On a broad basis, the principal orientations in eating are to include or exclude meat and meat products from the diet, although some adopt a smorgasbord approach. Meat eaters often do not have any particular preference for the animals and birds chosen for food, unless this choice is regulated by religious taboos. Within this group of eaters, we have the interesting group that adheres rather enthusiastically to the Mediterranean diet. By this we understand that a limited amount of red meat is eaten, small to moderate consumption of dairy products takes place, and there is moderate to high fish consumption. Fat intake is mainly in the form of monounsaturated fats and is represented primarily by olive oil. The diet is high in carbohydrates and fiber and has antioxidants and other helpful plant chemicals represented (we will look at these in the next section). Wine (red) is an integral part of the Mediterranean diet. The traditional Asian diet is also of scientific interest. In this diet, complex carbohydrates, mainly in the form of rice, are dominant. Seafood and limited intake of fats are characteristic, as is the mostly vegetable base to the diet. Large amounts of green and black tea are consumed.[93]

The contrasting group of people is vegetarian. In the broadest sense this includes those who supplement a plant-based diet with dairy products, eggs, and fish. Where fish and other meats occasionally are added to a basic plant diet, the individuals may be called flexitarians. Or, if animal protein is regularly added in small amounts, they have been termed vegivores. In a more restrictive sense, those who use only food from plant sources are known as vegans. There are many variations encountered under the last grouping, but we need to refer only to those who choose a macrobiotic lifestyle. This group accepts a vegan lifestyle in which the food choices are highly restricted.[94]

There are several particularly beneficial dietary components associated with a vegetarian lifestyle. These can be highlighted as follows:[95]

a)   *High fiber.* Plant-based diets contain a selection of natural items rich in fiber. This has the generally accepted effect of reducing the risk of colon and rectal cancer rates.

b)   *Phytochemicals.* These non-nutrient plant chemicals have reached the headlines on account of their possible benefits for health. Some fascinating information is emerging that we will take up in a subsequent chapter. A diet rich in vegetables and fruits contains an extensive range of plant-associated chemicals.

c)   *Unsaturated fats.* An outstanding benefit of a plant-based diet is that it is rich in unsaturated fats. Plant oils, except coconut and palm kernel oil, are less saturated than animal-derived oils. One of the benefits is that a vegetarian diet lowers blood pressure and the risk of heart disease.

From the above comments, it should be apparent that even choosing the correct balance of building blocks for the construction of body cells is not sufficient to ensure optimal health.

Some additional concerns are mentioned in the following section.

Diet and Health

There are many fads and fancies surrounding questions of eating and good health. Today there is a vast amount of knowledge concerning health readily available and free.[96] The advice is to act from sound knowledge. We might add a note of warning. The Internet is full of information from various sources. However, it is to verifiable knowledge that we should direct our attention. This usually comes from institutions and groups devoted to the scientific method that involves rigorous experimentation and sound statistical analysis. Findings that are approaching the truth are repeatable. This means that we find a number of qualified practitioners reaching the same conclusions. I give one additional warning about the scientific method. Science is progressive. This means that all conclusions are tentative and subject to revision as new information comes to light. This should not disturb us, as this is exactly how we operate in real life when we are assessing what a new employee or a new acquaintance is like.

One of the more interesting findings of science in recent years is that the wisdom held by a number of ancient cultures has merit.

One of the more interesting findings of science in recent years is that the wisdom held by a number of ancient cultures has merit. One group I have in mind limited the use of meat and avoided the eating of blood (kosher killed meat). Some may wish to question such advice, but they should first wait to see the evidence. There also are two regional groups of people who have done rather well through limiting the intake of meat: Mediterranean and Asian. I will briefly mention some of the advantages of these dietary approaches in relation to certain diseases. First, I will commence with cancer.

Cancer

Scientists inform us that at least 35 percent of cancers can be prevented by attention to diet.[97] We will reap the consequences of our actions, whether in the physical or spiritual realms. For example, one of the consequences of overeating on a regular basis is obesity. This leads to an increased risk of a variety of cancers, including breast, prostate, endometrial, colon, and gall bladder, and other diseases through changes in hormone balance and to substances released from fat cells.[98] The lifespan will be shortened by our choices.

People who eat little meat manage to reduce the incidence of cancer on account of their choice. Meat eating is associated with an increased risk of colorectal cancer. Those who reduce meat intake generally increase the intake of plant-derived food components (with their protective chemicals), which accounts in part for protection. However, more specific information has come from a number of studies and most recently from human volunteers. Red meat has a rich supply of blood proteins and heme (myoglobin and hemoglobin) associated with it. One suggestion is that these proteins react with other chemicals present in the digestive tract that are formed under the conditions normally present there and further that heme stimulates the formation of cancer-producing substances. As a result, carcinogens such as nitrosoamines are made. Now, red meat is a much richer source of iron containing proteins (particularly myoglobin) than white meat, thus potentially explaining its strong association with increased cancer risk.

The risk of contracting colorectal cancer is increased by 12–17 percent per 100 grams of all meat or red meat consumed per day.

Processed meats also fit into the same risk category as red meats. It has been estimated by one group of researchers that the risk of contracting colorectal cancer is increased by 12–17 percent per 100 grams of all meat or red meat consumed per day; the risk is much higher for processed meats.[99] While these estimates have been questioned, The World Cancer Research Fund recommends that those eating red meat should restrict intake to less than 500 grams per week. They noted that an individual eating a serving of red or processed meat daily for 40 years had a 20 percent increased risk of developing colon cancer. Individuals prone to eating meats cooked at high temperatures (grilling, frying, and barbecuing) increase their exposure to substances that are cancer producing, as do those who eat meats that are salted, smoked, and treated with nitrous compounds.[100] The American College of Nutrition recently recommended that avoiding red meat has advantages beyond cancer risk reduction and encompasses diabetes, hypertension, and cardiovascular disease. They went on to observe that all the nutrients contained in these products could be gained from plant-based diets.[101]

How this fits into the idea of stability or homeostasis may be reasonably simple to explain. It has been suggested that the nitroso-compounds interfere with cellular stability and cause stress. In practical terms this means that the dangerous compounds identified above are able to cause a lesion in the genetic material (DNA), injuring it and its ability to operate with fidelity. As a consequence, the cell's physiological stability is lost and cancer may develop.[102]

Those in some ancient societies who took the advice of their sages seriously and restricted the intake of blood through eating kosher or similarly killed meat (some still do this—Jewish, Islamic, and some Christian groups) reaped health advantages, although they did not understand the reason (Leviticus 7:26).[103] The Bible is very clear about the inadvisability of eating foods containing blood. It is significant to note that this advice has come to us most recently from the first church council held in the Christian era (Acts 15:20). The shedding of blood, whether of humans or animals, is a result of the entrance of sin into the world (Genesis 3:21; 4:8–12). It should not stretch our imagination to think that the continual shedding of blood is not in God's plan.

In the Jewish economy, God's advice about the eating of blood was followed rather scrupulously, and today we are familiar with kosher meats. The process of producing kosher meats involves draining the carcass of blood, removing prohibited fats and certain veins, arteries, and nerves. In order to remove the blood still in the meat, it is soaked in salted water.[104] It is interesting to note that the carcass of animals such as sheep, pigs, and cattle, when slaughtered by traditional methods, actually contains around 50 percent of the original blood, with different muscles retaining more or less.[105] Hence, the process of preparing kosher meat is rather detailed.

We have noted already that many cancers are preventable. Exercise, weight management, and dietary changes are the keys to reducing risk. The advice is quite simple. We can increase our risk of developing cancer by eating lots of grills, barbequed, fried, pickled, and salted products and saturated animal fats and certain animal proteins. Among proteins, dairy products are considered particularly unhelpful in excess by some

scientists. For one thing, prostate cancer risk appears to be increased by high calcium, dairy-based intake diets.[106] Eating fruits, vegetables, and whole grains will decrease our risk. The cruciferous vegetables (cabbage, broccoli, kale, etc.) that are used commonly among Chinese populations provide protection against colon and prostate cancers, but a considerable number of other plants contain anti-cancer substances too. Soybeans contain several protective chemicals that are thought to account for the lower incidence of breast, prostate, and colorectal cancers in Asia. Now there are other polyphenol-type dietary components from fruits and vegetables that are being studied extensively for their ability to moderate the risks of cancer development. Fiber is another important component of plant-based products. It reduces stool transit time, and it has other beneficial functions. It has a particularly protective effect against colon cancer.[107]

This means that whole grains, fruits, and vegetables are beneficial in reducing the risk of gastro-intestinal cancer. Those reading the signs will avoid saturated fats together with other damaging materials and will give increased attention to natural products from the plant kingdom.[108]

Not only is colorectal cancer incidence reduced by fruits and vegetables, but the benefits are also seen in a lowering of lung, mouth, esophagus, and stomach cancer. This is indeed good news, and it gets better if regular physical activity is engaged in.[109]

Highlight: *Diets high in whole grains, fruits, and vegetables and low in meats, particularly red meat, promote cancer avoidance.*

Diabetes

The question may be asked legitimately, why is diabetes increasing so rapidly in our society? Diabetes is both a significant and growing public health interest in many places, particularly

Western nations, but the trend is seen in the Asia-Pacific region as well. There is a veritable epidemic in China and India. Diabetes (especially type 2 or non-insulin dependent diabetes) can be prevented or delayed through managing the risk factors. Keeping the body fat down and being physically active are the key strategies to adopt in order to prevent its development and to successfully treat it. Evidence suggests, too, that the intake of high levels of saturated fats during pregnancy compromises the future health of the baby. Avoiding excessive levels of saturated fats, highly refined foods, and realizing the value of grains and vegetables are important parts of any successful strategy.[110] God's initial plans for the human race included both participating in regular exercise and eating exclusively of fresh foods. Refined foods were not available (Genesis 1:29; 2:15; 3:18–19), making us certain that diabetes was unknown to early humans.

Diabetes increases the risk of heart disease, kidney dysfunction, blindness, and limb amputation. In type 2 diabetes blood glucose levels are elevated because the body cells do not respond normally to insulin. This hormone allows cells to use glucose to obtain their energy, but in type 2 diabetes glucose is not absorbed properly by the cells.[111]

Blood glucose control is made simpler by eating starchy, high fiber carbohydrates. Simple carbohydrates found in honey, soft drinks, sweets, biscuits, fruit drinks, and the like are out! We do well not to overload on proteins, and we definitely need to keep fats under control. It is wise to eat less and not to eat in front of the television. The advice is to say 'no' to fatty and sugary foods and second helpings! In other words, take control of your eating.[112]

Remember that vegetarians are at less risk of developing diabetes in contrast to meat eaters. In fact, there is a positive relationship between how much red meat and processed meat that is eaten and diabetes.[113] The suspect compounds are called advanced glycation end products (formed from interactions between sugars and amino groups on proteins and the like). These are found naturally in some foods, especially those high in protein and fats of animal origin. Cooking at high temperatures and dry heat ensures they are present in especially high amounts. There is also a gentle warning that caffeine intake in the form of coffee, tea, and cola drinks is a risk factor for type 2 diabetes and could exacerbate it in those already showing symptoms of the disease.[114]

The key to understanding blood glucose levels resides in understanding the glycemic index. This index is a system of classifying carbohydrates in terms of how quickly and strongly they cause blood sugar to rise. The higher the index value, the more care we need to exercise in the use of the food item, for regular strong blood glucose spikes are bad for our health. The glycemic index is raised by eating highly processed products. The more finely ground a product, the higher its value on the index. The good news is that we can choose our foods wisely by consulting the index on the Internet.[115] The general advice for those without this facility is to use minimally processed foods and largely avoid sugar and soft drinks. We might carefully note that some fruits are rich in natural sugars but do not raise blood sugar levels as strongly as some starchy foods; how the sugar is packaged in the food is thus important. Dietary fiber (soluble and insoluble forms) plays important functions in human health. Soluble fiber particularly appears to convert carbohydrates into a slow release form that lowers the insulin required for uptake into tissues. This and other factors contribute to reducing the risk of diabetes and other diseases.[116]

I mention a simple but important fact here. We should not fall into a common trap and think that simple sugars such as fructose and glucose found in honey are any less damaging than cane sugar (sucrose) or other simple sugars when taken in excess. All simple sugars are problematic when taken in excess. The scientific community understands that there is a tendency to overweight and other problems through foods and drinks loaded with simple sugars.

Highlights:
1. *Avoidance of sugary drinks and foods and instead eating starchy, high fiber carbohydrates lowers the risk of diabetes.*

2. *Vegetarians are at less risk than meat eaters of contracting diabetes.*

Heart Disease

Keeping our hearts ticking longer is a question that concerns many people. Atherosclerosis is largely a preventable disease. The key to this is to maintain vessel system health by keeping it in a state of stability. A large intake of fatty foods is not a good choice. Surprisingly, this was understood by one ancient people group (Jewish) where the advice was given to avoid eating animal fat (Leviticus 7:23). At a rather later time (600 BC), the Indian physician Charaka specifically noted the link between heart disease, overeating, lack of exercise, and stress.[117]

The relationship between heart disease and fat intake is not free from dispute in scientific circles. A number of studies have shown that the risk of heart disease is reduced by limiting the intake of fatty foods containing saturated fats and replacing them with unsaturated fat and at the same time taking on a diet high in fiber and micronutrients from fruits and vegetables. Particular classes of saturated fatty acids have different effects so that sweeping statements can no longer be made about saturated versus unsaturated fats. The jury is still out on the intake of coconut and palm products, which are exceptional in the plant kingdom in that they contain a high proportion of saturated fats.[118]

The following information should help readers to form an opinion.

Combining a Western diet with the intake of all but small quantities of coconut products could be problematic.

The richest source of saturated fats is the oil from these plants. The composition of palm oil differs considerably from coconut oil.[119] The latter oil has a high percentage of fatty acids that increase good cholesterol (HDL), although it contains some fatty acids that raise levels of low-density lipoproteins (LDL). The overall effect in populations eating significant amounts of coconut products differ depending on the other components of their diet. For example, the Kitavans (Melanesia) have a low incidence of coronary heart disease (CHD) whereas groups from Sri Lanka have a relatively high incidence. The difference between the populations is thought to be attributable to the high fish, fruits, and vegetables consumption among the Melanesians. Complex interactions occur among nutrient components, and sociological factors also come into play. This means that combining a Western diet with the intake of all but small quantities of coconut products could be problematic, especially if coconut oil is chosen as the primary food item.[120] Coconut milk and flesh contain a lower percentage of fats than coconut oil.

The risks of consuming palm oil with its high levels of saturated fatty acid has not been fully assessed, but it appears to be relatively risk free as long as there is not an excess level of dietary cholesterol present in the diet.[121] The oil when freshly prepared contains powerful antioxidants, which gives a clue to its relatively neutral impact on heart disease. However, when the oil is repeatedly reheated (a common practice in Asia) some of the beneficial properties are lost, allowing its use to increase the risk of heart disease, at least in animal models.[122] When all the data are considered, there are perhaps better options than using palm oil, as demonstrated in animal experiments. Extra virgin oil actually decreased disease lesions when fed to mice (diet mimicked Western), whereas palm oil fed animals showed accelerated lesion formation.[123]

If we are in a position to lower our cholesterol levels, this will be beneficial in reducing the risk of vascular and heart disease. The heart-damage-risk-marker cholesterol (some is needed by the body) can be lowered by reducing the intake of eggs, meat, and full fat dairy products (includes cheese). Fish is exceptional in that it contains beneficial omega-3 polyunsaturated fatty acids (good plant sources are found in nuts and beans) but on the other hand it still contains cholesterol in reasonable quantities.[124] When we speak of reducing the level of one risk factor in the diet, careful readers will be aware that substitutes should contribute to the trend toward healthful eating. For example, reduction in saturated fats should not be associated with a compensatory increase in refined carbohydrates.[125]

While talking about meat in the diet, it recently has been suggested that the tendency for red meat to increase the risk of heart disease may be due to additional substances found in abundance in this food item. The first or these is carnitine. It is in relatively high concentrations in red meat, especially lamb and dairy products. This substance is changed by microbes in the body. The changed circulating substances actually slow the removal of artery clogging material. Hence, white meats are items of first choice, for they contain less carnitine than red meat. The body produces all the carnitine it needs to carry out its functions of transporting fatty acids, so we do not need to worry about including it in the diet.[126] Then there are the advanced glycation end products found in abundance in foods rich in protein and fats, especially those of animal origin.

Their presence has been associated with diseases such as atherosclerosis and chronic kidney disease. These findings constitute additional incentive to reduce one's dependence on animal-based foods.[127]

Other dietary components contribute to heart health. An important component of the Mediterranean diet is olive oil. In fact, it is the main fatty acid component of such a diet. This mono-unsaturated fatty acid (major component is oleic acid) exerts a number of health benefits and some of these are on account of the presence of anti-oxidant agents (polyphenols). Olive oil decreases the levels of low-density lipoproteins (LDL) and total cholesterol. High-density lipoproteins (HDL or good) cholesterol levels remain unchanged.[128] Many benefits have been attributed to including this oil (particularly high quality lines) in the diet. These include decreasing the risk of atherosclerosis and the risk of contracting certain cancers. Additional benefits have been claimed for those who have diabetes, rheumatoid arthritis, gastric ulcers, and gall bladder problems.[129]

The good news is that the effects of our poor choices can be reversed through exercise, stress management, and dietary decisions that reduce fats. We might consider the use of polyunsaturated fats (e.g., corn, safflower, and soy) or monounsaturated oils (e.g., canola, olive, and peanut). If we include foods rich in vitamin E (seeds, nuts, and vegetable oils), carotenoids (organic pigments), and flavonoids (compounds that exert estrogenic actions on animals), then we reduce the formation of dangerous types of low-density lipoproteins. Flavonoids are present particularly in fresh, ripe plant foods and berries, and there are more present in the peel than the pulp. The yellow, orange, and red pigments associated with fruits and vegetables are carotenoid pigments. This means we are advised to eat plenty of fresh fruits and vegetables and regularly use nuts if we wish to lower our risk of heart disease. The soybean and its products are especially valuable in lowering blood cholesterol levels.[130]

Highlights:

1. *Fatty foods, particularly those laden with saturated fats, can increase the risk of heart disease.*

2. *Polyunsaturated fats (typically plant sources) and many plant foods have beneficial effects on heart health.*

Maintaining cardiovascular health is not only about diet. Exercise and other forms of physical activity are also significant. It has been estimated that about half of the population in industrialized countries places themselves at increased risk of premature death from heart and other diseases on account of lack of physical activity. Health benefits are to be reaped through moderate levels of physical activity undertaken on a regular basis. The death rate drops if we walk 1.6 kilometers (1 mile) per day. Further benefit is observed after 4.8 kilometers (3 miles). Recommendations other than walking involve participating in moderate or vigorous activity three to five days per week. High intensity activity capable of causing sweating, for even short periods of time, is particularly beneficial.[131]

Half of the population in industrialized countries places themselves at increased risk of premature death from heart and other diseases on account of lack of physical activity.

Asthma and Allergies

The increase in prevalence of asthma and allergic diseases in urbanized, Western countries has been linked provisionally to the increased intake of processed foods. Adoption of a diet favoring high intake of whole grains, fruits, vegetables, and minimally processed foods has been associated with a reduced incidence of these conditions. Intake of fruit exerted a particularly noticeable positive impact on health maintenance.[132]

Gastric Ulcers and Cancer

The question sometimes arises: Do fiery spices harm the body? It should not surprise us that the answer is that fiery spices do damage the body. They are irritants according to common experience, and this is substantiated by detailed scientific evidence. Spices such as pepper, chili, mustard, and cinnamon irritate the stomach or in other words make it difficult for the cells to operate in a balanced manner. When we combine irritation through this means with a stressful lifestyle, then the way is opened to damaging the mucosal lining in the stomach. This makes the organ susceptible to ulcer formation. Scientific research suggests that eating highly seasoned food (e.g., high consumption of chili and other hot spices) on a regular basis is not a wise choice for a number of reasons. Too many associations have been found between the incidence of different kinds of cancer and the intake of very spicy foods to make their consumption advisable, although it is fair to say that not all studies support this line of thought.[133]

Highlights:

1. *The intake of fast foods is associated with a higher incidence of asthma and allergies.*

2. *Highly seasoned foods, when continually eaten, are thought to exert a deleterious effect on health.*

Infectious Diseases

The relationship between consumption of meat and their products and increased risk of microbial-associated food poisoning is a well-established scientific principle. The foods most frequently implicated in Western countries are of animal origin (meat, poultry, milk, eggs, and their products).[134] Microorganisms involved upset the homeostatic balance in the body and cause disease and sometimes death. Bacteria and viruses are commonly involved in poisoning episodes, with their significance varying between countries. One reasonably frequent disease (yersiniosis) is caused by an organism found commonly in animal reservoirs of which pigs are the primary source of human infection. It is frequently the case with this disease and other animal-associated illnesses that raw or poorly cooked products are utilized. Other causes are the improper handling of products.[135]

Well before the modern era when science had established clear linkages between microbes and disease, protection was provided from another source. God originally provided plant-based foods for human consumption, but this was modified later on account of the need to overcome food shortages (Genesis 1:29; 9:3). Not all animals are considered the same; the Bible makes a distinction between animal groups. Some it terms clean and others unclean and when sea creatures are considered, the understanding is that those with fins and scales are edible and the others are not to be used (Leviticus 11:2–7, 9–12, 13–19). Many dismiss these distinctions as having no basis, but before this is done, perhaps a little background to some Bible verses should be considered.

I will attempt to explain why some groups still find the distinction has meaning. First, when Noah was instructed to make provision for the conservation of created species in the ark he had constructed at the time of the great flood, God had already made the distinction among animals (Genesis 7:2). This was well before the Jewish race came into existence and before the Mosaic laws were established. Moses highlighted the distinction among the animals again in very clear statements (Leviticus 11).

The apostles knew and reverenced these provisions as illustrated by Peter's horror when God instructed him to "kill and eat" all manner of animals (Acts 10:10–16). This dramatic vision was given to Peter for the purpose of impressing upon him that all peoples are invited to join God's kingdom. It had nothing to do with eating preferences (Acts 10:28). We come finally to the instruction of the apostle Paul to "let no one judge you in food or in drink" (Colossians 2:16). This is taken by some as proof positive that all food is equal before God, as affirmed by a number of commentators. Others see this instruction as referring to the eating of food and drink offered to idols, which is a subject often spoken about in Paul's writings (Romans 14; 1 Corinthians 8). It is well known that pagan priests carried out a vigorous trade in meat taken from animals offered as sacrifices.

Now, if we suppose for a moment that there is something in the distinction made by some Bible verses about the advisability of eating certain food items, is there any scientific information available to give it credibility? In other words, there is no need to lose valuable information on account of the fact that the meaning of the verses cited above has been made unclear.

Some suggestions can be made to help us here; for some they may be conclusive and for others they may not be so convincing. First, some scaleless fish—skates, sharks, shellfish, and crabs—are poisonous. This is particularly noted with the puffer fish and its relatives, certain crabs, octopuses, and other animals that carry the extremely toxic tetrodotoxin. Shellfish often have been associated with poisoning episodes (five types identified) and allergic reactions. In fact, they are one of the leading causes of food allergies.[136]

Of more general significance, filter-feeding shellfish/bivalves are well-known carriers of organisms capable of causing human disease. They concentrate the disease organisms in their flesh. This means that raw and lightly steamed seafood taken from coastal waters is associated consistently with disease. It has been estimated that eating such food causes around 40,000 deaths annually and a similar number of cases of long-term disability, such as chronic liver damage.[137]

Secondly, the most reasonable view is that, in general, the animals considered unsuitable for food by various people groups (unclean) are those that feed on filthy foods, dead animals, and the like (carnivores/scavengers).[138] If we take the pig as an example, it is often fed on scraps, which has its own consequences. In an article written by the well-known Australian scientist Professor Gold-smid, some years ago, he relates "pork … is the source of a number of serious human diseases, including toxoplasmosis, trichinosis, and pork tapeworm …."[139] The incidence of these diseases differs around the world. The pork tapeworm is still widespread in Central and South America, Asia, and Africa and affects millions. It may cause epileptic fits and even death, since the parasite may lodge in the brain besides the eyes and muscles.[140] Trichinosis is a disease caused by a parasitic worm that is widespread and of some significance in Central and South America, Europe, Asia, and China. The pig, other mammals, birds, and reptiles may be infected. Humans, horses, and pigs are the most significant hosts. Pigs readily acquire the parasite on account of their propensity to eat infected carrion, rats, and the like. Larvae present in incompletely cooked meat are released in the intestines. The worm undergoes a number of changes, migrates through the body in the circulatory system and lodges in skeletal muscle fibers.[141] The disease may be fatal in rare instances. Mild symptoms involve fever, headache, gastrointestinal discomfit, muscle soreness, inflammation and ocular pain, and disturbed vision.[142]

Large and small outbreaks of the disease have been recorded in some countries, such as the Christian communities of Lebanon and Syria on account of consuming wild boar. No such outbreaks were recorded among the Muslims for the simple reason that the Koran forbids the use of pork, just as the Bible does. This is the general pattern in other Muslim countries as well (other meats may be infected so some outbreaks have been recorded) and where Jewish communities are found. Rather spectacular outbreaks have been recorded in the Arctic following eating of bears, walruses, and other animals that are considered unclean.[143] With this background information, it is not surprising that the prophet Isaiah had some rather sharp words to say about eating the flesh of swine and unclean animals (Isaiah 65:3, 4). Those who understand God's Word as it reads, as do Seventh-day Adventists, take the advice of Moses and Isaiah seriously and avoid unclean foods.

One of the diseases carried by many animals is toxoplasmosis, which affects approximately 30 percent of the world's population. This disease is caused by a rather common parasite that is often found in domestic cats and rodents, particularly in the tropics. The parasite is of interest to all pregnant mothers or those infected just before pregnancy. Infection by this parasite can cause stillbirth and may lead to a variety of complications including blindness and brain damage. It may be consumed in undercooked meat from sheep, cattle, and pigs and is widespread in cat feces.

Food, utensils, or hands coming in contact with raw meat or contaminated soil may also become cross-contaminated. The disease is of unusual current interest among scientists because it apparently adversely affects the reaction times in people who have come into contact with it (this is definitely of interest to motorists). There is also some evidence that it is a risk factor for schizophrenia and depression. The continuing research is worth following.[144]

Highlights:

1. *Infectious diseases are carried by animal foods much more commonly than plant-based foods.*

2. *Some highly damaging disease organisms are carried by so-called "unclean meats" and others by "clean" meats.*

Hormones and Antibiotics in Animal-based Food

The use of animal products from genetically altered animals is a cause for considerable debate. The use of engineered bovine growth hormones to increase milk production is used extensively in North America. While U.S. authorities are unwilling to admit to unwanted effects, others are not so ready to follow. There are reasons to believe that there could be links with the elevated levels of growth factors present in milk from treated cows and the occurrence of various cancers in humans (particularly on account of the higher levels of insulin-like growth factors present and its ability to predispose to cancer) besides some reported multiple adverse effects on animal health. Additional issues have been anticipated in alterations to the developmental pattern in humans, the possibility of consumption of these products being responsible for the early onset of puberty, and for contributing to the rise in chronic diseases. All these questions are asked legitimately besides those that arise from contaminating the environment with these hormones and their possible effects on the life events of animals in aquatic systems.[145]

There are reasons to believe that there could be links with the elevated levels of growth factors present in milk...and the occurrence of various cancers in humans

---

Meanwhile the European Union rejected the practice of using substances having a hormonal action for the purpose of promoting farm animal growth and objected to imports of such products (includes natural and engineered hormones). The commission considers that the data available do not allow a realistic estimate of the risks involved, which includes the possibility of some hormones acting as carcinogens. They consider that caution is the preferable course of action.[146] This caution is particularly merited as previous experience among Puerto Rican girls, who consumed meat contaminated with a chemical that mimicked hormones (diethyl stilbestrol), showed precocious signs of early puberty. This hormone was used to fatten cattle and poultry. It also was used to prevent miscarriages in women. Later it was shown to be a carcinogen, and its use has now been discontinued.[147]

Another question causing debate is the use of antibiotics in livestock production. They are commonly used in order to stimulate weight gain, improve efficiency in food use, and improve general animal health.[148] While it is undoubtedly true that these benefits are seen, there is the danger that antibiotic resistant strains of pathogenic bacteria will be selected in animals through the continual application of these antibiotics.[149] When these bacteria are transferred to humans in food, disease may develop under selected conditions and the organisms may be unresponsive to related antibiotics prescribed to control them. The dangers are fully recognized in some countries, and the European Union has a limited use policy. This limited use policy is not followed by all countries, which leaves open the possibility of antibiotic resistant strains developing widely and with it the lessening of effective control measures.[150] These modern developments in animal husbandry stand as evidence that a plant-based diet has many advantages.

Highlights:

1. *Treating animals with growth hormones or modifying them genetically to promote growth can conceivably have unwanted effects on humans and the environment.*

2. *The use of antibiotics in agriculture can assist in antibiotic resistant strains emerging in the human population.*

Genetic Modification of Foods and Health

Another question of considerable interest with plant-based diets is to what extent genetic engineered plants are used and what dangers they pose.

Some plants are poorly adapted to absorb nutrients from the soil and they may be modified genetically to allow them to do so again. In other situations, such as in some parts of Asia, Africa, the Caribbean, and Latin America, vitamin A deficiency affects millions of children with blindness (250 million under five). Here the use of genetically modified golden rice or modified bananas could prevent vitamin A deficiency. These projects are still in the evaluation phase. If varieties are made available for local farming, immediate and immense health benefits would be delivered. Modifying plants to give higher levels of unsaturated fatty acids or vitamin content (A, B, C, and E) are some of the avenues being exploited. Additional research is being carried out to invent plant varieties that are less allergenic (e.g., peanuts, cereals, etc.).[151]

Without getting into the detailed arguments for and against the use of such foods, we can record that the use of genetically modified food in the United States over a number of years has not turned up any significant human health problems, although claims have been made particularly relating to plant health. This is of potential concern as plants form the basis of most food chains. It is well known that plants are widely grown that have been engineered to contain a gene that renders them resistant to the herbicide glyphosate (Roundup®). The utilization of this technology allows weeds to be controlled while leaving the plants containing the gene unaffected. Limited information exists to suggest that sometimes herbicide treated resistant crops appear to be less effective in absorbing nutrients and more susceptible to selected soil diseases. Claims about human and animal health effects have not been proven, yet some of the preliminary evidence suggests all may not be well.[152]

Caution is probably the best advice on account of some potential problems that have been identified. For example, food items have been found contaminated by genetically modified plant products meant for the pharmaceutical trade (pharma plants) or for animal feed. Such mistakes could have serious implications for peoples' health. In addition, the transfer of genetic information from cells containing novel combinations of DNA to bacteria in the human gut is a source of guarded concern.[153] Genetically changed plants have the ability to modify communities of organisms in the soil environment in which they grow; the seriousness of this impact is debated.[154] In passing, it might be noted, however, that plants modified by traditional plant breeding programs sometimes lead to health problems such as induction of skin rashes and allergic reactions. Similar issues might occasionally be expected with genetically modified plants. This means that great care needs to be exercised in the development and approval processes for such products.[155]

Highlight: Genetic modification of food either by classical breeding techniques or modern methods can be useful, but some modifications may be dangerous. Caution is advised.

I now turn from the cautionary tale about plants and focus on the really good news.

Can Foods Modify Us Genetically?

This question may seem strange, and, indeed, if it had been asked several decades ago, one would have been ridiculed. Today, the answer is yes: foods can modify the expression of our genes and influence how we respond to environmental risk factors. The chemical substances that surround our heritable material (DNA) are able to modify the expression of genes in a cell. These substances are contributed to by our diet. The research on epigenetics suggests that obesity, diabetes, cancer, and some immune disorders are influenced by the prenatal diet.[156] This means that what we eat, we are, and what our mothers ate influences our subsequent life history.

Foods of particular interest are folic acid, vitamin B_{12}, and some bioactive substances from plants—garlic, broccoli, soybean, and others. The development of the early embryo can be adversely affected by high fat diets and alcohol consumption. This field of endeavor is relatively new and is based on animal studies, so knowledge applicable to humans is limited. However, it is beyond dispute that the bodily functions of animals and how an animal responds to risk factors or assaults by disease organisms is influenced by what they eat.[157] This means that we, and also our progeny, are affected by our dietary choices. Thus choose carefully!

Functional Foods and Health

Some plant foods are termed functional because they contain active components that provide benefits beyond that contained in their basic nutrients. Protection against cardiovascular disease is claimed for some foods such as soybeans, oats, psyllium, flaxseed, garlic, tea, fish, grapes, nuts, and additive-enhanced (plant sterol/stanol added) margarines. When eaten consistently and in adequate amounts, these foods may decrease disease risk.[158] Clearly, all the evidence has not been gathered. We notice that the scientific community claims they "may" reduce disease. However, one natural product that has received considerable attention is the grape.

Grape products have been used since antiquity as medications. For example, we notice the advice given by the apostle Paul to Timothy: "No longer drink only water, but use a little wine for the sake of your stomach and your frequent ailments" (1 Timothy 5:23, ESV). The medication being spoken about was probably similar to that noted by Aristotle, Pliny. and others. Commonly such medication involved the use of unfermented grape juice mixed with water.[159] This advice leads us to consider a similar debate that has exploded in the news media.

The current debate in some circles centers on the benefits of special plant chemicals in food items that provide health benefits. Red wine has been shown to contain a component (resveratrol) that reduces the risk of heart disease and, in animal experiments, has been shown to be a cancer preventative. Now the truth of the matter is that the same component is present in fresh grape juice and more than seventy species of plants including mulberries and peanuts.[160] Naturally, these facts are not commonly made known, especially by the wine industry. However, one must acknowledge that the red grape (skin) is a very good source of the compound. Resveratrol stimulates the production of special enzymes and activates biochemical pathways, thus protecting selected cells from damage. In this manner cell health and longevity are preserved. The protective effects of a range of plant chemicals (phytochemicals), including resveratrol, can shield individuals from neurodegenerative diseases as well.[161] In all the discussion, we should not forget that restriction in calorie intake is the greatest boon to longevity, as it diminishes the deleterious effects of reactive chemicals produced in the body and has positive influences on the genes for longevity.[162]

Restriction in calorie intake is the greatest boon to longevity.

Wine also contains flavonoids (particularly a group of substances called procyanidins) that offer protective effects against a range of diseases including heart disease.[163] These components are also available in apples, various berries, plums, and other food items,[164] so the health benefits of red wine now comes into better perspective. One quickly comes to the realization that an individual does not have to resort to taking alcoholic drinks in order to obtain the benefits of components held in the grape. Then it must be remembered that many alcoholic drinks are not derived from this fruit.

In fact, the American Heart Association warns nondrinkers not to start in the hope they will realize health benefits. The benefits of alcohol consumption in protecting drinkers against cardiovascular disease may be due to the antioxidants contained in the beverages and to lifestyle factors rather than to the alcohol itself.[165] And the National Cancer Institute considers that alcohol consumption increases the risk of colorectal cancer generally and breast cancer in women (7 to 12 percent). Such risk is associated with a consumption increase of less than one drink (10 grams of alcohol) per day.[166] Overall, it has been noted that "no major health organization has ever called for encouraging nondrinkers to start consuming alcohol for their health."[167] This is particularly relevant in light of the most recent research that brings the "hypothesized cardioprotective effect of alcohol into question."[168]

Our initial comments have been about grapes and their products. However, there are many other antioxidant-containing products and other protective chemicals found in fruits and vegetables. Some of these protective chemicals reduce blood clotting and reduce the effect of inflammatory agents. One of the ways functional foods act is through removing from circulation reactive oxygen and nitrogen molecules. These molecules are produced continually, but more are generated under certain disease conditions and where oxygen is used at high rates (vigorous work or exercise). They are very reactive and destroy body cell components, so removing the excess is beneficial. The food components able to do this are called antioxidants. These are commonly of plant origin. It is believed that antioxidants may aid in the prevention of cancer, atherosclerosis, stroke, rheumatoid arthritis, neurodegeneration, and diabetes.[169] I will comment on several additional antioxidant components that have been investigated.

The medical profession has been fascinated with the Mediterranean type diet and its positive contribution to good health. Somewhat belatedly, the Asian diet (largely plant based) is also now receiving more attention from the scientific community.[170] One component commonly found in Asian diets is the soybean. Intake of traditional soy foods (not concentrates or pills) reduces breast cancer risk as well as improves bone health. The benefit found by eating this product apparently resides in the isoflavonoids contained in it—principally genistein and daidzein. Many of the known benefits relate to their antioxidant properties.[171] Genistein can exert protective effects against prostate and breast cancers.[172]

A prominent food component in the Mediterranean diet is the tomato and its products. These contain lycopene (an antioxidant). A number of studies have related lycopene levels with a reduction in risk for coronary heart disease and various cancers. This effect is noted particularly when cooked and processed products are used in preference to the raw tomatoes. This is on account of the bioavailability of lycopene being increased by processing. Wild plants found in the Mediterranean region, such as wild artichoke, also help to protect the heart.[173]

The evidence is becoming quite strong in favor of the positive effects of antioxidants; in reality these products aid in maintaining cellular homeostasis. Now, the natural occurring antioxidants mentioned specifically above are better than their synthetic counterparts. This is on account of other protective chemicals being present in the natural product; overdoses also are unlikely to occur when natural sources of plant chemicals are used.[174]

Highlights:
1. *Many protective chemicals are found in plant-based foods.*
2. *The protective chemicals are best taken in their natural state.*

Mineral and Vitamin Supplements

Normally, eating a variety of plant products will ensure an adequate mineral and vitamin supply. In the previous chapter we considered special needs groups and discovered that there are several circumstances where care is needed in order to maintain cellular stability and whole body health.

Degenerative diseases such as aging, cognitive decline, and poor functioning of the immune system can be moderated by ensuring that there is adequate intake of vitamins, minerals, amino acids, and fatty acids. There is one hypothesis currently advocated that the most telling impact is made early in life. In later life we reap the rewards of early malnutrition episodes (before birth) or subsequent neglect.[175]

Many countries fortify salt with iodine in an attempt to prevent iodine deficiency developing with its associated physical and mental retardation. Upwards to a billion people are at risk from iodine deficiency as a consequence of inadequate supplies in the soil in which the plants are grown.

In some areas of China, selenium supplementation is also needed to overcome endemic heart disease problems for similar reasons.[176] Today's earth is not the same as when it was first created, if we follow the Christian story of origins (Genesis 2:15–17; 3:17–19).

Fruits and vegetables are a rich source of most vitamins when they are fresh. They are significant to the robust functioning of the immune system. The aging process is not kind to the human body, and the function of the immune system declines. Now this system is vital if we are to fight off infectious disease agents, and its ability to do this is influenced by nutrition. Deficiencies in a whole range of amino acids, fatty acids, vitamins, and minerals can weaken its function. The good news is that enhanced levels of vitamin E and zinc can improve the function of the immune system. Studies have suggested that vitamin E supplementation in the aging population may be beneficial. However, those on anticoagulant therapy or suffering from coagulation defects must proceed under medical instruction.[177]

There is one vitamin that those dedicated to a vegetarian lifestyle need to think about carefully. This is vitamin B_{12}. Those on a vegan diet (no meat, milk, eggs, or cheese) often have low serum levels of this vitamin. Occasionally lacto-ovo vegetarians (eat dairy products and eggs) also have low serum levels. Fortified or supplements are necessary for vegans in order for acceptable levels to be maintained in the body.[178] The bioavailability of vitamin B_{12} differs considerably. This vitamin, when found in meat (fish, sheep, chicken), is 42–66 percent available, whereas from eggs it is less than 9 percent available. Dried green and purple lavers (nori—genus *Porphyra*) and button mushrooms (*Agaricus bisporus*) contain amounts of the vitamin together with a variable quantity being found in some fermented products.[179] However, expert opinion is that those eating vegetable based diets exclusively need to be aware of B_{12}

deficiency issues and eat reliable sources of the vitamin.

It would be hard to find anyone who would argue against the advantages of adding the vitamin folic acid to cereals in order to reduce the occurrence of spina bifida. However, the same enthusiasm does not extend to the addition of a range of other additives to food. For example, the eating of beta-carotene in isolation from food may increase the risk of cancer.[180] Then we have the possibility that people may overdose on certain additives if added to foods because they have a weakness for a fortified food item—such as biscuits. The natural way is the safest way. Other special groups of people may need supplements to improve their health, but the craze about vitamins sweeping many countries has its downside. Excessive intake can be dangerous. Vitamins taken in excess, particularly the fat soluble ones (A, D, E, and K), can be toxic or interfere with proper body functioning.[181]

Highlights:

1. *Plants may be deficient in some minerals growing in mineral depleted soils.*

2. *Supplementation of the diet with folic acid and vitamin B_{12} is merited in the pregnant and aging.*

Restricting Calorific Intake

Behaving in a temperate manner involves self-control, which is wisdom contained in many philosophies both past and present (1 Corinthians 9:25).[182] This advice has its own benefits when it comes to eating behavior. It has been found that if we restrict our caloric intake our life will be extended.[183] When we become obese, our adipose tissues do not have the ability to secrete hormones that allow the maintenance of cell stability.[184] Restricting our calorific intake is important to cellular as well as whole body health, such as

cardiovascular disease and degeneration of the nervous system.[185]

Girls that come to puberty at an early age have a much higher risk of breast cancer than those who arrive at this state at a later age.

A puzzling feature noted in girls in Western nations is that they are reaching puberty at a progressively earlier age than previously recorded. The explanation is far from simple with genetics, physical activity, nutrition, family conflict, disrupting chemicals, and other factors being proposed.[186] One theory is that body fat is responsible, for puberty occurs later in girls with a lower percentage of body fat. It is thought that fat cells are involved in signaling the brain to secrete hormones that raise estrogen levels.[187] This may have implications for the development of breast cancer later in life. In fact, girls that come to puberty at an early age (twelve or younger) have a much higher risk of breast cancer than those who arrive at this state at a later age. The risk is reduced by 9 percent for every year that puberty is delayed. The risk is also apparent in girls who experience peak growth early (taller early) and even greater in those who reach puberty early. The influence of early age puberty on cancer risk is due presumably to the increased length of exposure of susceptible cells to ovarian hormones on account of both the greater number of cycles of hormone exposure experienced and the longer time to first pregnancy. It is suggested that restricting calorie intake and maintaining physical activity are essential to reducing cancer risk.[188]

Highlight: Restricting calorific intake has many benefits that involve whole body health. The risk of breast cancer in women is reduced and life is extended.

Guiding Principles and Practical Suggestions

1. The ability to maintain the body in a balanced and stable state is related to dietary choices.

2. The Mediterranean and Asian diets promote health and traditionally are high in complex carbohydrates and fiber. Since there are liberal quantities of fruits and vegetables included in some of these diets, good supplies of protective chemicals are guaranteed. In practical terms little meat is consumed in these diets.

3. Our health status is influenced by our dietary choices as illustrated by the dietary factors, predisposing individuals to cancer, atherosclerosis, diabetes, asthma, and allergic conditions. Overconsumption of foods, particularly rich foods (high sugar and fats), and a failure to exercise predisposes one to cancer and heart disease. Whole grains and legumes eaten at every meal aid in resisting cancer and heart disease.

4. Eating largely of red and cured meats and dairy products will lead to poorer health outcomes.[189] A liberal intake of saturated fats (solid at room temperature) as opposed to unsaturated fats (liquid at room temperature) also predisposes to disease.

5. Highly refined and sugary foods and drinks, fats, and a failure to exercise are sure aids in the development of type 2 diabetes. Sugary drinks are best avoided. Water and unsweetened drinks are the best choice for continued health.

6. Animal-based foods place individuals at a greater risk of contracting selected infectious diseases of microbial origin. All foods, irrespective of their origin, should be refrigerated when processed or kept at high temperature (60°C) until eaten. Cross contamination between animal products and plant-based products should be avoided. Good hygiene should be practiced at all times in order to prevent contamination of foods from fecal sources.

7. Animal-based foods containing growth hormones and antibiotics pose a potential health hazard, which has been shown rather conclusively with the latter group of contaminants.

8. Genetically modified foods have both real and potential dangers and their use must be considered carefully. Ultimately, we are what we eat.

9. Many foods of plant origin contain active components that provide benefits beyond that contained in their basic nutrients. They provide protection against some of the modern diseases found in society. It is generally considered unwise to isolate the active protective agents and consume them in concentrated form. Eating whole foods are much superior to consuming isolated food-derived chemicals.

10. Maintaining a balanced supply of minerals and vitamins assists in maintaining the homeostatic state and whole body health. Fruits and vegetables are a rich source of most vitamins when they are fresh. A modern trend in some societies is to consume vitamins and selected minerals in tablet form on a regular basis. Generally this is unnecessary if a fresh supply of fruits and vegetables is eaten. Cooking or storing these items leads to a loss of activity. Vitamins are retained best where foods are

fresh or minimally processed. Minerals such as iron (needed to prevent anemia) are found in legumes, tofu, and green leafy vegetables, such as spinach and bok choy, dried apricots, nuts, and seeds.

11. Eating organic food reduces the damaging effects of unhelpful chemicals in our foods.

12. Eating in moderation is guaranteed to bring better health and to increase life expectancy.

Chapter 4

Maintaining Nerve Pathways

Humans have shown an ability to find biologically active substances in nature for thousands of years. The Chinese knew about cannabis almost three thousand years before Christ and the Persians popularized hashish.[190] Some of the oldest archaeological sites also contain evidence that humans used mind-altering substances. Recent excavations at a site in modern day Turkmenistan have revealed a structure used for religious activities dating from around four centuries BC. At this place, there are altars that held the sacred fire and mind-altering drink, haoma, that were part of the religion of Zoroaster. The trance inducing drink (hallucinogenic) was taken so that the priests could contact the spirit world. In Central Asia the use of cannabis is clearly outlined by the historian Herodotus in ceremonies associated with burials among the Scythians, presumably because it gave rise to a trance like state of euphoria. The well-known use of opium in this region has been brought to a new emphasis by the recent history of Afghanistan. This highly addictive substance has a long history of use on account of its ability to induce hallucinations and a dreamlike state. It even was used in ancient Egypt in order to stop crying children.[191]

The use of stimulants in China goes even further back, perhaps five thousand years. There the shrubby plant ephedra was used to treat asthma and other respiratory problems, and it is still used in herbal medicinal drinks today. This substance came over into Western medicine in an altered form where it appeared in the original common cold anticongestant Sudafed. In sufficient amounts the active ingredient, pseudoephedrine, and its derivatives (amphetamines) stimulate the central nervous system and produce a euphoric state and, on account of this quality, was used by Native Americans and others.[192] There are many other historical records of the use of mind-altering drugs by peoples of various countries.[193] Today, there are marginal subcultures in almost every society that use such substances. In mainstream cultures, the use of alcohol, with its much milder effects, is almost universal. Caffeinated products are the most popular form of drug taking behavior in the world.[194]

Many biologically active substances are found in plant products where they perform essential functions. Some of these (bioamines—organic compounds containing nitrogen) affect the blood vessels or nervous system in various ways. Not all the effects are beneficial, and some substances are positively dangerous when taken in quantity.[195] This means that manufactured products containing "natural" ingredients should be considered carefully before unreservedly recommending their liberal use.

Highlight: Many biologically active and mind-altering substances have been discovered. Most of these do not contribute positively to temperate living or good health.

The use of drugs in their various forms is not the only human activity that influences health and clear thinking. Intemperate eating behavior has reached plague proportions in some cultures, but it is not a modern phenomenon. The ancients were enticed by the pleasures of eating. It is recorded that Claudius Caesar not only enjoyed drinking excessively, but he never left a party without gorging himself.[196] I mention so-called addictive eating here to reflect popular opinion. Scientific opinion suggests that in some individuals the intake of sweets, fats, and other foods can have a druglike effect on the body, which strengthens the idea that there may be food addictions. It has been discovered that the neurotransmitters in the brain associated with food addictions are the same as with addictions in general.[197]

Brain Function and Behavior

The brain is an amazing organ that has the power to think and generate emotions. Other organs cannot accomplish these functions. For many years the difference noted between the brain and other organs of the body led some Western philosophers to imagine that there was a great divide between the body and the mind. The distinction is no longer held. It now is realized that the brain is an organ in which complex electrochemical interactions occur. Changes in our behavior can be related to changes in chemical and electrical signals. Being mentally ill can be explained in the same terms. The mind and other body parts influence each other dramatically so that disturbances in one affect the other. Changes occurring in an organ of the body, such as the liver, affect the mind and sadness and anxiety generated in the mind affects the whole body. This means that the well-being of one part is intertwined with the other (1 Corinthians 12:12–25).[198]

Addictive drugs upset the stable state of the body and lead to various levels of dysfunction.[199] Each drug of abuse exerts its immediate effects on the nervous system using different molecular targets. This is on account of the great differences found in the active chemical carried by each drug that is responsible for the addiction. As the mode of action of drugs became more clearly understood, it was recognized that physical dependency on drugs is largely separate from addiction. The latter term refers to a compulsive seeking for a drug. It is now understood that clients may relapse into drug taking after many years of abstinence. This can be explained by the fact that selected cells adapt to drug exposure by undergoing permanent molecular and morphological changes. This means that the brain circuitry is changed through repeated exposure to addictive drugs.[200]

Highlight: The mind and body exert effects on each other so that changes and disturbances in one organ have significant influences on other body organs. Addictive drugs may lead to permanent changes in the brain.

Clearly the changes in the mind also influence other body functions. I will look at several habit-forming drugs that may influence behavior and influence health adversely.

Lifestyle Choices and Health

The adverse effects of some of our recreational and other activities have become apparent in recent years. There is now an almost universal appreciation of the link between lung cancer and smoking and a grudging admission that the use of cannabis is even more devastating. This association of smoking with lung cancer development and reduced lung function is so firmly established that involuntary smoking, through inhaling tobacco smoke produced by others, has also become a focus of concern in some countries.[201] The attitude of good living people toward habit-forming behavior, such as the use of tobacco or cannabis, falls into the same category as for narcotics.[202]

The debate about the milder drugs has reached new territory with the coming of highly sophisticated imaging machines that monitor brain activity. Alcohol has been the most widely used social drug throughout history with half of the adults in the Western world choosing to use it.[203] Moderate use is associated in some studies with a reduction in the risk of cardiovascular disease, stroke, and dementia (but see our discussion later). However, the smartness of even moderate use is being increasingly questioned following links being established between alcohol consumption and the

risk of certain cancers, diabetes, and other conditions.

It is interesting to note that the Cancer Council of Australia indicates that "any level of alcohol consumption increases the risk of developing an alcohol-related cancer," although it is fair to say that the more one drinks the greater the risk. However, the professional body recommends that the best course of action in order to reduce risk is to "avoid alcohol altogether," for the very simple reason that ethanol (present in all alcoholic drinks) is a group 1 carcinogen. This means that it has a proven ability to predispose to various cancers.[204] Serious studies have shown that less than one drink a day can significantly increase the risk of breast cancer in women, leading some to say that no level of alcohol consumption is safe. Alcohol appears to act as a cumulative carcinogen and maybe a tumor-promoter as well.[205]

Alcohol appears to act as a cumulative carcinogen and maybe a tumor-promoter as well.

The occurrence of binge drinking episodes among the young has introduced a new dimension of concern. It has been estimated that seven million American youth in the age bracket twelve to twenty binge drink at least once a month [binge drinking is considered to be four drinks (women) and five drinks (men) over two hours]. The possible effect of these excessive drinking bouts on mental capacity is frightening if we take the results of animal experiments into consideration. The risk of brain damage and dementia are increased. This is in addition to increasing the risk of breast cancer. Then there is a dramatic rise in injury to the liver and the possibility of epigenetic alterations—that is, gene expression is changed by exposure to alcohol. In animal experiments, as little as one day's exposure to high levels of alcohol exposure is sufficient to damage the brain.[206]

The young brain is more susceptible to alcohol damage than older brain tissue, and animal experiments suggest that repeated exposure to alcohol disrupts normal development. Binge drinking in rat models suggests by extension that a single episode in humans could cause degeneration of neural tissues leading to learning and memory impairment. In fact, in humans the volume of the hippocampus, which is the part of the brain associated with learning and memory, has been shown to be reduced in young individuals given to alcohol abuse. It was found that these individuals were also poorer on visual and memory tests than those shown in a comparable group of young adults not given to binge drinking. Similar drinking among pregnant mothers is especially damaging to the developing brain of the fetus, which subsequently leads to cognitive and behavioral defects in their children.[207]

Some further comment is merited on the reported positive effects of light to moderate alcohol consumption in reducing the risks of cardiovascular disease, stroke, and dementia. The first thing to note is that not all research indicates a positive effect between light-moderate alcohol consumption and reduction of cardiovascular disease risks; in fact, some even have noted a negative effect on hypertension. Gender and race may be significant in determining the outcome. With stroke, the effects of light to moderate consumption again varies among studies, so that consumption may reduce the risk, be without impact, or may be deleterious for some population groups and for one type of stroke. The positive effects of alcohol consumption often are associated with the use of red wine. It contains many substances (polyphenols, such as resveratrol, quercetin, etc.) other than alcohol (ethanol) that exert biological effects. One of the important functions of the polyphenols is to inhibit platelet aggregation, an effect found with alcohol too. In fact, some believe that these polyphenols are protective independent of alcohol, which is given credibility by the observation that the beneficial effects on heart health can be achieved by de-alcoholized wine. Wines differ widely in polyphenol content depending on the source and processing. An interesting observation is that olive oil also has protective qualities as do other plant foods high in polyphenols, such as berries, chocolate, walnuts, peanuts, and other fruits and vegetables.[208] This means we have ready access to safe alternatives that are enjoyable and are able to protect our health.

Similarly, stroke risk reduction can be achieved by means other than alcohol consumption. Dietary choices that include high intakes of fruits and vegetables are bound to assist in the control of hypertension and reduce the risk of stroke. These diseases are common worldwide. This means that dietary modifications that include at least 600 grams of fruits and vegetables a day would reduce the global disease burden by an estimated 1.8 percent.[209]

Finally, commenting on dementia, one group of Italian experts has summarized the available research results on alcohol consumption and cognitive decline by stating that the data are inconsistent and that those who do not drink presently should not be encouraged to do so. Their recommendations are that "it is reasonable to encourage the consumption of adequate fatty fish and foods rich in vitamins and antioxidant nutrients as a part of general dietary recommendations." They go on to say, after discussing the use of alcohol: "no data suggest to supplement the diet with additional pharmacological treatment,"[210] which put simply means—eat what God has provided from the natural world. This is very close to the position taken by the prophet Daniel recorded in

Daniel 1. All those who are seeking to live a holy life will avoid partaking of alcoholic drinks.

Highlights:
1. *Smoking cigarettes or using cannabis has many adverse effects on health.*
2. *Alcohol use and misuse among the young and pregnant is particularly damaging.*
3. *Beneficial influences of light-moderate alcohol intake can be achieved through eating fatty fish and a diet rich in fruits and vegetables.*

The French Paradox

Much scientific data has been accumulated to indicate that high saturated fatty acid intake is not compatible with maintaining heart health. However, in France there is a low incidence of coronary heart disease although the population has a high intake of saturated fat and cholesterol. In seeking to explain this paradox, several theories have been explored.

The first line of investigation followed the high but regular consumption of wine among the French and suggested that alcohol consumption was the beneficial agent through raising high-density lipoproteins. However, the disturbing feature was that high-density lipoproteins are no higher in France than in other countries. In trying to resolve this enigma, it is considered possible that alcohol may be one factor that contributes to protection from coronary heart disease through reducing platelet aggregation.[211] Another protective component is resveratrol. However, this compound (trans form) is found in other sources, such as in black grapes and their products and at high levels in the well-known Itadori tea (produced from *Polygonum cuspidatum*). Furthermore, the latter product has been used for centuries in Japan and China as a remedy for heart disease and stroke.[212]

Investigators have also considered that other components of the wine exert significant protective effects. Components of grape (red) skins and the fruits and vegetables characteristic of the Mediterranean diet may be responsible for the protection offered, in addition to physical activity and attitude. This means that diets rich in fruits and vegetables and where regular leisure time exercise is practiced are likely to deliver beneficial outcomes as far as heart disease is concerned.[213] Indeed, in a group of subjects who had suffered a heart attack, dietary interventions were made to determine if recurrences might be reduced. A substantial reduction in coronary events was achieved by supplying a comparatively rich supply of linolenic acid (supplied in special margarine—canola based and similar to olive oil) by increasing oleic acid and by reducing linoleic acid. The protective effect of antioxidants and vitamin C in the intake of fruits, vegetables, and wine also accounted for the protection of these subjects. Whether the red wine exerted a specific protective effect could not be assessed as the controls drank as much as the experimental group!

In another study along similar lines conducted with south Asians at high risk of cardiovascular disease, increasing the quantities of fruits and vegetables and maintaining a high level of usage of whole grains, pulses, and mustard oils (rich in n-3 fatty acids such as alpha linolenic acid) were found to be protective. Intake of alcohol was permitted, but discouraged, as was smoking. Exercise and mental relaxation were encouraged. The investigations pointed to the possibility that n-3 fatty acids supplied by mustard or soybean oils, walnuts, whole grains, and vegetables may be a good alternative to fish or fish oil supplements.[214] In all these studies, it is significant to note the role of attitude toward food in achieving health outcomes. Stress and pleasure exert their own effects on both the cardiovascular and immune systems. The reality is that when country differences in diseases are compared then genetic, environmental, diet, psychological variables, and the level of medical care all play their part.[215]

While all studies have their critics, the difficulties in performing such experiments in an ethical manner are quite challenging. Trivializing the complexity of the issues involved and arguing against the advances of science do not aid achieving welcome community health outcomes. Some final words may be said about the effects of alcohol on memory-related tasks. Alcohol has selective effects on transmitter systems in the brain so as to alter the activity of some signal receptors. Adolescents are more sensitive to memory and learning impairment, which is measurable after two to three drinks.[216] No wonder that the Bible records that Daniel and his friends refused to drink wine but chose water instead. Their memory superiority over their contemporaries was outstanding (Daniel 1:8–20). Their example is worth emulating.

Alcohol has selective effects on transmitter systems in the brain so as to alter the activity of some signal receptors.

Highlights:

1. *A number of components of the diet may have moderating effects on potentially harmful elements present.*

2. *Harmful dietary components, such as the group 1 carcinogen alcohol, with its mixed useful and non-useful effects can be substituted for by non-harmful components to perform the same useful functions.*

Living Drug Free

Some of the strongest motivation to avoid narcotics and habit-forming drugs come from those steeped in moral and ethical lore that holds that humanity was created in the image of a personal, creator God. Consumption of alcoholic drinks is considered a major sin or unwholesome act by devoted Muslim believers[217] and this is also the view held by selected Christian communities.[218] The attitude of careful Bible readers toward alcoholic beverages is colored by the advice of King Solomon, reportedly the wisest man living in ancient times. He informs us from experience that both wine and strong drinks are best left alone. He likened the adverse effects of alcoholic beverages on health to the bite of poisonous snakes. He considered that in order to have clear thinking people in charge of the affairs of the nation should abstain from wine and strong drink (Proverbs 23:31, 32). His best advice is given in the following words: "Wine is a mocker and beer a brawler; whoever is led astray by them is not wise" (Proverbs 20:1, NIV).

The same advice goes for everyone else who wishes to think clearly and discern between right and wrong. The Jewish prophet Isaiah was adamant that those who use "intoxicating drink" could not fulfill the demands of public office or bring glory to the supreme God (Isaiah 28:5–8). King Lemuel's mother adds her words of wisdom in Proverbs (31:4, 5) by saying that those in charge of the affairs of state should leave "intoxicating drink" alone. This is good advice.

The link of drink to crime need hardly be mentioned.[219] Alcohol's effects on the physical and psychological well-being of the individual are well documented. The acute effects of alcoholism are reversible in the absence of alcohol consumption, but chronic alcoholism leads to many changes including morphologic alterations mainly in the liver and stomach. Such changes increase the risk of cancer (hepatocellular carcinoma).[220]

Many in the Christian confession picture early Christians as advocating and using fermented wine in religious and other activities. This view is probably uncontestable.[221] However, historians and classical writers have left sufficient evidence to allow strong statements to be made about both the practice and methods of preservation of both fruits and unfermented grape juice from ancient times. This means that it is possible to make more than one interpretation of the ancient texts, as they may often be read to refer to both fermented and unfermented wine.[222] Since fermentation is used as a symbol of sin in the Christian scriptures and Jesus lived a life without fault, believers seeking to follow His ways neither use nor advise others to partake of fermented beverages, for they believe they are called to follow Jesus' example explicitly (1 Peter 2:21). The soundness of this reasoning perhaps becomes evident when we look at the provisions made by God for those under His special care.

In the Exodus experience when the children of Israel were taken from Egyptian bondage into the land of Canaan, God provided them with water (Exodus 17:6). After all, those seeking peak performances in the spiritual life should perhaps not come behind endurance sports people. One authority speaking about this group said: "One would hope that endurance athletes would be among those inclined not to drink alcohol."[223] Now, the apostle Paul likens those who are living as Christians in an evil world as athletes (1 Corinthians 9:24–27). Our attitude toward alcoholic drinks should be the same as that recommended for endurance athletes.

In Christian literature there is a substantial basis for refusing to take or deal in narcotics.

Other habit-forming drugs are similarly considered out of bounds by the groups mentioned previously. In Christian literature there is a substantial basis for refusing to take or deal in narcotics. This is on account of the example left by Jesus who refused gall and vinegar offered to reduce the agony inflicted on Him by His enemies (Matthew 27:34). This refusal functioned to keep His mind clear. Some, even among Jewish sources, believe that the gall offered Jesus was a narcotic preparation obtained from the opium poppy. The Christian Scriptures' attitude toward narcotics is exceedingly clear. The word sometimes translated as sorcerer in the New Testament is derived from the Greek word *pharmakeus* (Galatians 5:20; Revelation 9:21; 21:8; 22:15). This also can legitimately be applied to the pushing of drugs.[224] We find that Islamic sources and some Buddhist groups are equally clear about the unfortunate results of using narcotics.[225] The scientific and sociological evidence available on the deadly effects of drugs such as heroin and cocaine do not need to be listed since they are so well known. Their adverse effects are seen in the unborn as well.[226]

Highlights:

1. *The moral guidelines of a number of philosophies (Buddhist, Christian, and Islam) argue for moderation and/or abstinence when dealing with alcoholic beverages.*

2. *The use of other habit-forming drugs (narcotics) is considered unwholesome by these groups.*

Christian believers have the strongest reason for rejecting the use of habit-forming drugs in that they hold that the body is to be kept from being "defiled." This means they consider that God created them for the express purpose of bringing honor to His reputation as pure and wholesome individuals. As a consequence, they choose not to undertake any activity that will lead to cell injury and perhaps hasten their death (Exodus 20:13; 1 Corinthians 3:16, 17; 10:31).

Jesus' provision of wine at the wedding at Cana might reasonably be interpreted to indicate that He provided grape juice rather than the fermented product (John 2:3, 7–10), for the host was well able to discern the superiority of the product near the end of the feast (verse 10). In addition, leaven is a symbol of sin (yeast in this case), and Christ was without sin (1 Corinthians 5:6–8). This means that to attribute the use of alcoholic beverages to Christ is neither a reasonable or consistent proposition (Note: in Matthew 26:29 Jesus was careful to make all aware that the communion beverage was the "fruit of the vine" or grape juice). He would hardly have participated in such an activity when His brief was to overcome a very smart individual (Satan) who had already deceived and misled the human race in addition to many of the angels in heaven (Romans 5:12; Revelation 12:7–9). As He was the maker of the delicate human machinery (John 1:1–3), it is hardly a tenable argument to suggest He advocated damaging it by providing addictive material to His followers.

In times of difficulty, God has promised His servants that their bread and water will be sure (Isaiah 33:16), and in the new earth pure water will be available (Revelation 22:1). One might reasonably argue that Christ followed healthful principles, for His emphasis on difficult issues was to point His hearers back to the beginning—Eden (Matthew 19:4–6).

Highlight: *There is no credibility to the argument that Christ drank alcoholic beverages or provided them for others to drink.*

In the next section I will give some information on the significance of water usage.

Water Usage

Water is essential for life. It is the liquid used by the animal kingdom to satisfy its needs, as designed by the Creator (Genesis 2:10; Numbers 20:8). It is an essential nutrient, comprising 55–60 percent of total body weight in adults.[227] Humans alone have invented other ways to satisfy thirst. In contrast to pure water, it is probably true to say that no other hydrating fluid is its equal, although this is not to infer that some of humanity's inventions are not helpful and enjoyable. Pure water has the advantage that it has no adverse effects.

I have reminded readers previously that God designed the human body and provided water to satisfy the requirements of this complex piece of biological machinery (Exodus 17:6; Numbers 20:5, 8). However, it is not possible to meet ideals at all times and in all places. For example, in many cities of the world, water in the tap is neither pure nor safe chemically or microbiologically.[228] Even some bottled water may be unsafe from a chemical perspective.[229] Those seeking to function optimally and to use the most healthful source of water will need to consult those with local and regional expertise. Where such sources cannot be found, alternative safe hydrating liquids need to be sought.

A fascinating study of the relationship between fatal coronary heart disease and intake of water, involving a large study group, has shown clearly the advisability of drinking water. Those drinking five to more glasses daily substantially lowered their risks. When some other fluids were used, the advantage was not observed. This outcome possibly is on account of caffeinated drinks being diuretic and soda drinks causing a movement of fluid from the blood vessels. While the study had its limitations, the importance of maintaining blood fluidity is undeniable. The Food and Nutrition Board of the Institute of Medicine gives recommended daily dietary intakes of water as 3.8 liters for men and 2.9 liters for women.[230]

Water has other impacts on general health. Dehydration alters the balance of electrolytes (salts, acids, and bases) in the body, leading to difficulties in making saliva and maintaining skin elasticity. Headaches may develop, and the individual is predisposed to constipation, kidney stones, urinary infection, and the risk of pressure ulcers developing (hospital situation). There is some evidence that cognitive function is impaired in the elderly who are dehydrated and the risk of falling is increased. The effects of dehydration are noted particularly in the elderly, but are not absent in other age brackets either.[231] All this seems a good incentive to drink more water.

Highlight: Water is an ideal hydrating agent. Its consistent and abundant use lowers the risk of coronary heart and other diseases and conditions.

In the next section I will give some information on how selected drugs bring about cell alteration and injury.

Cell Injury

Cells respond to chemical, physical, and other stimuli. Their response depends on the stimulus type, duration, and severity and the genetic makeup of the cells involved. Cells may be injured by contact with stimuli. This may lead to biochemical and functional abnormalities in key structures or processes, and this will impact the health of the individual. There are many agents that may cause cell injury. These range from chemical substances to dangerous microorganisms, from nutritional imbalances to physical agents and to aging.[232] However, we are particularly interested in providing information relevant to a group of selected chemical agents.

I will commence with a note on nicotine. Individuals smoke in order to relax when they are tense and waken them when drowsy, for nicotine stimulates the reflexes beyond conscious control (autonomic). There are receptors in the brain that respond to nicotine, and they increase in number following chronic use. This is really an adaptive response that leads to tolerance. The individual becomes addicted by nicotine and develops

dependency. A number of substances present in the smoke, such as tars and other irritants, are carcinogenic. This means that they interfere with the normal functioning of the cell. It is held that 90 percent of lung cancers are associated with smoking. Then there are other diseases such as chronic bronchitis and coronary heart and vascular diseases that are strongly related to smoking activities.[233] Where smoking is common, strokes are also widespread, as noted particularly among China's teaming population of smokers.[234]

Marijuana (cannabis) use leads to equally damaging outcomes. Its use distorts the sensory perceptions and interferes with motor coordination, and its continued use leads to cognitive and psychomotor impairment and an inability to judge such things as speed, distance, and time. It is associated with the inhalation and retention of three times as much tar in the lungs compared with cigarette smoking. Similar carcinogens are inhaled as when cigarettes are smoked, but more of the damaging materials are inhaled and retained. This causes damage to both the heart and lungs. Airway passage diseases and risk of carcinomas are increased, and individuals with preexisting heart conditions are placed in additional danger.[235]

Highlight: Smoking tobacco and marijuana (cannabis) is addictive and highly injurious to health. A Christian with this knowledge would not trade in self-harm.

The most widely used category of drugs is the methylxanthine group, such as caffeine and theophylline. The former component is found in coffee, tea, and chocolate and the latter in coffee and tea. The major effects are on the central nervous system, which they stimulate with a consequent reduction of fatigue and an increase in concentration and thought. Increased formation of urine (diuresis) occurs, and the cardiac muscle is stimulated along with relaxation of smooth muscles.

Tolerance (decrease in pharmacological effect) and adaptation (cessation causes adverse effects) occur to a small extent.[236]

Those who eat abundantly of fruits and vegetables have other avenues of acquiring the helpful chemicals found in tea, coffee, and red wine.

The subject of coffee and health is far from simple. While there are apparently some health benefits, there is also a downside. Groups such as children, adolescents, the pregnant, the elderly, and those with hypertension may be more susceptible to the adverse effects of the cocktail of chemicals such drinks contain.[237] There is conflicting evidence on the performance of individuals on selected memory tasks following the intake of caffeine, which makes claims of improved memory as a generalization suspect.[238] The relationship between intake of tea and coffee and heart disease has been investigated in a number of studies. There definitely is uncertainty over the long-term role of coffee, with the clearest wisdom being to restrict intake. Green tea consumption is associated with a reduced risk of heart disease, ostensibly for the reason that antioxidants are increased in the plasma.[239] Tea (green or black) is a rich source of flavonoids. This group of compounds reduces the risk of cardiovascular disease.[240] It should occur to readers that those who eat abundantly of fruits and vegetables have other avenues of acquiring the helpful chemicals found in tea, coffee, and red wine,[241] which means the claims and counterclaims surrounding drinking these substances need not concern many. A little known downside of excessive tea consumption using inferior brands (green and black) is they can lead to fluoride-related bone diseases.[242]

A major impact of caffeine is on sleep regulation (through interfering with the adenosine pathway), which means that when caffeine is no longer taken the individual is prone to sleepiness. In an extensive study of Icelandic adolescents using caffeine drinks, data indicated that they also were prone to more anger and irritation.[243]

Energy drinks are also basically caffeine products and may contain up to two and even four times as much caffeine as is present in a can of Coke. These drinks are laden with sugar and contain other additives. Some alcoholic drinks are also being marketed that contain caffeine. The adverse effects associated with the consumption of these drinks are insomnia, nervousness, headache, and accelerated heart beat (tachycardia), and some caffeine-associated deaths have been recorded.[244] Then there is the suggestion that energy drinks provide a gateway to other forms of drug dependence.[245]

Highlight: *Caffeinated drinks have a downside. The modern craze with energy drinks is more problematic and may lead to other forms of dependency.*

Desires to feel good and to escape from or cope with the challenges of life are the main reasons why people take on drugs of various types. There are other ways in which we may seek to find relaxation and relief. In the next section I will look at several of these.

Relaxation and the Desire to Feel Good

When the body systems are functioning well, particularly the dopamine signaling system, we feel good. If the system is not functioning well, then some people may seek to gain control by taking drugs such as cocaine.[246] However, there are other ways in which we may seek enjoyment.

Life is meant to be enjoyed, and there are a variety of ways in which various societies have sought to facilitate this. An ancient and popular practice was to promote various forms of spectator sports. This form of relaxation is still popular. However, there is no substitute to actual participation in the sporting activities. There are several other well-known and widespread relaxation and coping practices that are worth commenting upon. These practices are particularly relevant in the stress-filled world in which we find ourselves. I will mention some here but many more are available. The principles generated from the few examples taken should serve to inform the more general view.

Revelry

One popular device that the young engage in, so as to relax and seek enjoyment, is some form of revelry. It is observed that revelry is associated with certain types of suggestive music and other activities that satisfy the basal lusts for which the human race is well known. History contains some graphic accounts of the excesses of past civilizations (Exodus 32:6, 7; Numbers 25:1–3; 8).[247] And we do not have to search far into our own culture to understand the violent, crude, lawless ideas that are promoted by some leisure activities. Attraction to alcohol, drugs, and sex are a sure outcome. This should not surprise us following the discovery that these activities all stimulate similar brain regions.[248] It is not only the Christian philosophy that advises against a fascination with and fixation on alcohol, drugs, and sex (1 John 2:15–17; Revelation 2:6).[249] These activities reflect negatively on the robustness of the philosophical ideas adopted and bring discredit on the corporate body. There is really no difficulty in supporting this view if the Bible is taken seriously (Romans 13:12–14; Galatians 5:19–25; 1 Thessalonians 4:3–5).

Eating

Enjoying food can be another form of relaxation. As the economic robustness of a society or of individuals improves, it seems almost inevitable that dietary changes will occur and that physical activity will be reduced, leading to poor outcomes.[250] It is observed in many parts of the world that major increases in caloric intake and dietary changes are taking place. The intake of edible oil, caloric sweeteners, and animal products have shown rapid increases. These changes have resulted in rising levels of cardiovascular and other diseases.[251] There is unassailable evidence that a diet that contains a minimum intake of meat and refined foods and includes a liberal intake of grains, nuts, vegetables, and fruits is beneficial to health. In any lifestyle choice, an intelligent understanding of nutritional and physiological issues is of fundamental importance.[252] Both calorie selection and calorie limitation contribute to good health.[253]

The idea of temperance or moderation is almost a forgotten idea. However, the Christian philosophy emphasizes this concept (Numbers 11:4, 32–34; 1 Corinthians 9:24–27; Philippians 3:17–20), but with variable compliance being observed among its practitioners. Moderation has to do with self-control, which is important to success in life. Children learn self-control as they understand and accept behavioral norms for themselves. Parents are able to transmit these values to their children more effectively if they are loving, warm, and careful to explain why a particular behavior is wrong and how it will affect others.[254]

Television Viewing

There are some relaxation activities that are commonly encountered that have unwanted and perhaps unanticipated effects. We refer to the widespread practice of spending long hours viewing television programs or other entertainment industry packages. What we think is influenced by what we hear, see, and feel. If we choose to fill our minds with violence and unkind speech and behavior, we are being conditioned to react to others in a manner that reflects our mental diet.

In the scientific world, there is really no information of substance to indicate otherwise. Antisocial behavior may be taught by the mass media (television, heavy metal music, music videos, etc.). Then there are the difficulties with sleep and obesity that flow from long hours spent in amusement. Those with vested interests in the products that saturate the modern media markets will argue against it having an adverse effect on human behavior, but virtually no one else will join this chorus.[255] Few would spend the vast amount in advertising if no results were forthcoming! If for no other reason, TV and video viewing (also games) for long hours should be discouraged in favor of involvement in exercise and creative activities. This is not to suggest that these modern devices cannot act as excellent educational tools or promote relaxation of a genuine healing kind, such as through humor or comedy.

It is a truism that what the mind dwells on will determine what the individual will be like. If children are taught cooperative activities and given toys that promote such behavior, there will be a good uptake of information and helpful, cooperative behavior will be the outcome.[256] This good advice was anticipated by a Christian writer from antiquity who said: "whatever is true, whatever is just, whatever is pure, whatever is lovely, whatever is gracious, if there is any excellence, if there is anything worthy of praise, think about these things" (Philippians 4:8, RSV; cf. Psalm 101:3).

Meditation

In today's stress-filled world, everyone needs both physical and mental rest. In addition, many religious movements advocate a form of meditation to gain inner peace or find rest for the mind. This has the added advantage of promoting physical calmness and good health.[257] The type of meditation that various groups promote differs. Eastern traditions (Buddhism, Hinduism, Jainism) use various practices involving posture, breathing, mantras, and regulating sensory inputs. In the meditative state generated by following some Eastern cultural traditions, the person focuses inwardly and avoids external stimulation or is open to suggestions coming to the mind without judgment (they are simply viewed in a detached way).[258]

> *Meditation is not a mind-emptying activity where mantras or other repetitive mental devices are used.*

Scripture advocates meditation in a quiet environment where the individual has uninterrupted opportunity to think on uplifting themes. These themes may involve considering scenes from the life of Christ or of faithful prophets and the experiences of persons showing great faith (Matthew 6:6).[259] Such meditation is not a mind-emptying activity where mantras or other repetitive mental devices are used. In this belief system it is understood that any activity that has elements of repetition of meaningless thoughts, sounds, visual images or which use repetitive devices such as beads (tactile repetition) run counter to the advice given in a parable by the greatest of the prophets, Christ. In this account the individual described is shown as emptying the house of the mind of everything but filling it with nothing. The final result was worse than the starting position (Matthew 12:43–45). In many forms of meditation advocated today, the mind is in a state similar to that experienced during hypnosis or subliminal suggestion (Matthew 6:7).[260] In such a relaxed mental condition, the mind is more receptive to ideas and thoughts that are self-generated and are clearly counter to the entire purpose of the experience from a Christian perspective.[261]

In contrast to the approaches usually associated with Eastern religions, the Christian experience follows the biblical model that is made abundantly clear by various Bible characters. King David gives the most extensive account of subjects worthy of thought (Psalms 1:2; 19) and the experience of others reinforces the belief that our thoughts are to be well directed (Joshua 1:8; 1 Samuel 1:10–13; Daniel 9:3–22). During prayer sessions our thoughts are directed to God in heaven (Matthew 6:9; cf. Exodus 35:4–9). In times of meditation, the Holy Spirit may impress our minds to follow a particular course of action. Rarely, God or His messengers speak to individuals. If this happens, it is at times of God's choosing, not at our command (Exodus 33:18–23; 1 Samuel 3:4–11; Acts 8:26, 27; 9:1–6), as indicated for contemplative prayer exercises.

The desire and ability to feel good cannot be achieved fully in the absence of a positive mental attitude. A positive approach to life and its problems is conducive to health. We can challenge our initial reaction to adversity. Rather than sinking down into despair, we might ask what we can do to make a difference. Challenge negative thoughts. A positive attitude to life is taught by the day-to-day responses that parents and teachers make in the presence of growing children. Irrespective of a poor beginning, a negative attitude may be changed by disputing our initial response to trying circumstances. If the initial response turns out to be accurate, think of ways to move forward. Often there are more ways of looking at issues than we first imagined, so that our initial response turns out to be groundless or only partially correct (cf. 1 Thessalonians 5:15–18).[262] We might gain courage from the attitude of individuals who are featured in the popular news media. It was the double amputee Oscar Pistorius (Paralympian gold medalist) who declared: "I don't see myself as disabled. There's nothing I can't do that able-bodied athletes can do."[263]

While speaking of reasoning and other mental activity, it has been found that high levels of mental activity are associated with a reduced risk of dementia, and this reduced risk was substantial for those who after retirement participated in rich mental activity[264] This is an outcome worth striving for as a result of our relaxation activities.

Highlight: Involvement in activities from spectator to active sports, enjoying food, watching educational and humorous audiovisual programs, meditating and the like can generate positive mental attitudes and relaxation that is essential for the maintenance of health in the complex world in which we live.

Guiding Principles and Practical Suggestions

1. Changes occurring in an organ of the body such as the liver affect the mind and sadness and anxiety generated in the mind affects the whole body. This means that the well-being of one part of the body is intertwined with the other.

2. Biologically active substances found in nature have been used for thousands of years. They may have a beneficial or deleterious effect on the nerve pathways and other body functions. Some bioactive substances are addictive. A form of addiction is found with foods. Those high in sugars and fats exert druglike effects much as described for substance dependency.

3. Addictive drugs upset the stability of the body and lead to various levels of dysfunction. Selected cells adapt to drug exposure by undergoing molecular and morphological changes. This means that the brain circuitry is changed through repeated exposure to addictive drugs. They alter a person's behavior for all time.

4. One agent that does not upset the stability of the body is water. Its consistent and abundant use lowers the risk of coronary heart disease.

5. Christian moral and ethical lore holds that humans were created in the image of God and clearly advises against the use of mind-altering drugs. Those who use intoxicating drink cannot faithfully fulfill the demands of public office or pass a noble legacy onto their offspring. Habit-forming drugs are injurious to health and destroy the body and interfere with the ability of the individual to bring honor to themselves, their families, their communities, or to the founder of the philosophy they accept as guiding their life.

6. The desire to feel good is honorable. Lasting feelings of well-being cannot be achieved by engaging in revelry or excessive behavior. Moderation is a good principle to adopt in all our living. The desire and ability to feel good cannot be achieved fully in the absence of a positive mental attitude. Challenging negative thoughts is a good strategy to adopt.

7. Feeling good involves rest of mind and body together with sensible eating and relaxation activities. Informed sociologists advise us to offer toys to infants that promote non-aggressive themes. This means television viewing, video games, and real games involving guns, tanks, and similar weapons that promote aggressive encounters should be eliminated from consideration.[265]

8. Meditation on themes that promote goodness and rich mental activity are beneficial to health, well-being, and the development of spirituality.

Chapter 5

The Earth Mourns

In the modern world, the place we choose to live is often something that we can change only marginally on account of the varied work assignments that we must undertake in order to earn a living. We are living in a fast moving world that is thrilled with the prospect of making wealth on the one hand and burdened with survival on the other. It is an overpopulated globe that we share in which wealth is unequally distributed. The end results of industrialization and intensive agricultural activity are all too evident in pollution of air, water, and soil and degradation of the environment. The earth is mourning under the weight of the abuse it is suffering from. The apostle Paul says it this way: "For we know that the whole creation groans and labors with birth pangs together until now" (Romans 8:22).

Tourist destinations that offer relaxation in an environment where the beauties of nature may be enjoyed away from the maddening crowd are attractive to many, and this helps to illustrate the frustration that some have come to associate with city living. Where the choice exists, many would choose a quieter, more secluded existence known for simplicity in living. In such an environment the works of God are evident and give powerful proof of His creatorship and grandeur (Romans 1:20).

In the following discussion I will examine some of the problems of city living identified in scientific circles and how this impacts our health.

Pollution

There is really no need to seek scientific evidence for pollution in general, for we can see and smell it. However, we are seeking to identify some of the more subtle effects. Several broad categories of pollutants are worth considering.

Heavy Metals and Radioactive Substances

A number of well-publicized episodes involving heavy metals and radioactive materials have been recorded over the last half century or more. Contamination of fish with mercury and rice with cadmium in Japan are perhaps the best known. Both events led to tragic results and human deaths. Similar tragedies followed, and still continue, after the Chernobyl nuclear reactor disaster in the Ukraine.[266]

Smoke, Vapors, and Airborne Particles

The debate over lung cancer and tobacco smoke and the long-term dramatic effects of exposure to asbestos dust are well known. These examples represent just a few of those available to show that exposure to smoke, certain vapors, and dusts, which are much more concentrated in urban environments, is something we should not allow to happen on a regular basis. Lung function and health suffer from such exposures (resulting in bronchitis and asthma), and one's lifespan may be reduced.[267]

Individuals may be exposed to both indoor and outdoor air pollution. Indoor exposure to tobacco smoke, wood smoke, and bioaerosols (small airborne particles that may contain microbes), dust mites, pet dander, and the like can cause eye irritation, inflammation of internal areas of the nose (rhinitis), and asthma. Outdoor pollution is generated by particles released by various human activities and exhaust and industrial gases released from motor vehicles and manufacturing processes. The lungs take the main impact of these irritants. Then there are the occupational exposures to various chemicals, gases, and solvents, which may have dramatic adverse effects.[268]

Nutrients and Wastes

On account of agricultural and industrial activities, large quantities of waste may be produced. This may be disposed into landfill sites or intentionally or unintentionally find its way into aquatic systems. To many individuals, this seems a good solution. Just two examples will illustrate the weakness of this practice. Let us take the common agricultural nitrogen fertilizers used to stimulate plant growth and improve crop yield. Excess nitrogen not used for plant growth finds its way into river systems. These water resources may be used for human consumption. The nitrogen in this water (nitrate) may be turned into a toxic material (nitrite) by the bacteria present naturally in the human intestines. This leads to loss of oxygen carry capacity by the blood because methemoglobin is produced in the blood rather than oxyhemoglobin, and the blood's oxygen carrying capacity is reduced. In severe situations death may occur. Even in the United States, millions of families consume water that contains levels of nitrate in excess of the Federal standard and worldwide there are many reports of community-owned wells with concentrations of nitrate greater than the suggested World Health Organization guideline.[269]

> *Even in the United States, millions of families consume water that contains levels of nitrate in excess of the Federal standard.*

Additional problems may arise if the pollutants moving into water systems come from sewage either of animal or human origin. Serious disease outbreaks can occur. The most celebrated example is perhaps the cholera outbreak in London some

150 years ago when physician John Snow was able to demonstrate that water contaminated by sewage at the Broad Street pump was the source of the raging outbreak. The episodes of waterborne diseases of fecal origin since then are too numerous to list. However, the recent earthquake (2010) in Haiti and the epidemic of cholera experienced there illustrates the devastating results of such pollution. Hundreds of thousands died.[270]

Pesticide and Other Residues in Food

Food is potentially exposed to uptake of heavy metals, dangerous chemical pollutants, and radioactive substances that may be present in the soil. Then, in order to increase the amount of marketable produce, a range of agents is often used to kill weeds, insects, and microbes. As a result of these activities, chemical residues may be found in our food. In some countries standards are set so that pollutants may not go beyond a certain level. For example, in order to aid in enforcing these standards, regular surveys are conducted in some countries.[271] However, this is not to say that individual food items always pass. In some developed countries, such as the United States, and particularly in developing countries, unsafe levels of residues are found in a proportion of foods consumed.[272]

Highlight: *Pollution of the environment through human activities is present in almost every place we choose to travel. Being informed about the nature of the pollutants helps us to avoid some of the adverse effects they have on health.*

Environmental Degradation

The environmental movement is gaining strength on account of both better education and the greater visibility of the effects of environmental abuse. While the philosophical base on which it rests is often found contrary to Christian thought,

some of the issues highlighted are worth noting. I will look at several aspects of degradation that may impact our health.

Soil Degradation Leading to Plant Deficiencies

Degradation of the land leads to a loss in soil structure, topsoil, and plant nutrients. The latter are either lost to the air (dust particles or gaseous materials) or water systems, such as runoff of nutrients from agricultural lands into rivers. Plants growing on these lands subsequently will have fewer nutrients available to build into their structures, and food derived from these areas will have a poorer balance of nutrients. People or animals feeding on these plants could, in theory, find it more difficult to obtain a balanced intake of nutrients. This type of outcome has been found with animals. Among the human population, it has been discovered that eating extensively of plant varieties able to more efficiently extract nutrients from soils reduces the chances of deficiency diseases developing.[273]

Air Quality

The poor quality of city air has long been known to cause health problems. Elevated lead levels have an adverse influence on the intelligence of children, and other pollutants have their own peculiar influences on health. Prenatal exposure to selected pollutants can also impact the intelligence of children years later.[274] Recent studies have suggested that selected vehicle exhaust hydrocarbons may even damage the DNA of the unborn child and adversely affect adult health. Unwanted effects on lung, heart, and brain function have been associated with inhalation of diesel exhaust fumes.[275] The reality of such pollution is all too evident to those approaching large cities by air. As an example of the magnitude of the issue, the World Health Organization has estimated that in 2012 approximately 3.7 million premature deaths occured worldwide as a consequence of outside urban air exceeding safety limits for pollution. Many cities are unsafe and some countries do not have regulations on air pollution. Indoor air pollution contributes to even more deaths, with over half of the world's population being at risk of inhaling particles arising from heating and cooking fires.[276]

3.7 million premature deaths occured worldwide as a consequence of outside urban air exceeding safety limits for pollution.

Water System Degradation

Ever since the industrial revolution in about 1760, water system degradation has been evident with the inevitable loss of plant and animal diversity from these systems. Some of the great rivers and lakes of the world have become infamous for this trend. We might think of the Thames, the Aral Sea, and the Great Lakes as examples. However, degradation need not be a death sentence, as found with the Thames, which is rebounding to health. The effects of such losses may be primarily considered as a loss of livelihood, habitat, beauty, and the ability to enjoy restful activities in a particular locale. However, there are more insidious effects—the increase in disease producing chemical agents in these systems and the alteration of animals still living there cannot be dismissed. Toxic chemicals have been found in the fish in contaminated areas and may exceed levels considered fit for human consumption. When all sources of water pollution are considered (fertilizers, pesticides, agricultural runoff, sewage, other biological waste, heavy metals, chemical, and industrial

wastes) nearly 2.5 billion people worldwide are thought to live without improved sanitation.[277]

Organisms capable of causing human and animal diseases are frequently found in polluted waters. Fecal material in particular is involved and as a consequence disease is transmitted. Fish and shellfish living in contaminated waters (fresh or saline) may be the vehicle for transmitting disease. This is particularly the case when raw fish are eaten and when shellfish are taken from waters contaminated with fecal material, such as might happen during heavy storm water runoff and flooding. Contaminated recreational waters may pose additional risks in that skin and wounds may be infected and aerosols containing pathogens may be inhaled. Microbes frequently may find their way into drinking water through animal and human waste contaminating the source. This may result in serious illness and sometimes death. Alternatively, if fields are irrigated with wastewater or fruits and vegetables are washed in water containing fecal material, all sorts of unwanted outcomes can be experienced.[278]

Space Degradation

Population pressures lead to various adverse outcomes that are all too evident; these include noise and visual challenges. Several aspects of the crowding problem and the resultant visual pollution and destruction of nature and health are worth considering briefly.

- Imagination and well-being – Small living spaces have an influence on the feeling of well-being and change human behavior. Crowding contributes to children's imagination being poorly challenged. It has been found that contact with the outdoors is beneficial to mental, emotional, and social health.[279] Crowding in the environment outside the living quarters also affects one's sense of well-being. Many who have walked the streets of large cities can attest to the sense of disorientation or oppression, loss of a caring attitude and frustration. And there are yet other parameters to this experience.[280] Cities can be the loneliest places. The disengagement of some of their inhabitants is evident for they are regularly wired up to electronic devices to shut out all else.

- Antisocial behavior – Crowding may facilitate antisocial behavior. In cities crowds commonly gather and such gatherings influence how a person will react. The identity of the individual is reduced so that individual consciousness is altered. In a crowd the rational faculties of the individual are lowered so that a crowd mentality is established. The emotional reactions of the individual are more intense so that they contemplate doing things that "their consciences would forbid and their ethics would condemn." People may also show a disregard for usual caution and become irrational and irresponsible. Indeed, some go even as far as to say that individuals immersed in a crowd event behave like individuals under hypnosis.[281] In smaller groupings, such as gangs, members are forced to commit crimes that many would not participate in if they were by themselves. Gangs are antisocial and violent by nature and flourish where favorable sociological factors are found, such as generally associated with cities (Genesis 19:4, 5).[282]

- Poor accommodation – When accommodation is at a premium, we find that landlords often are more interested in investment returns than with the

comfort of people in the premises. Consequently, the physical plant is allowed to deteriorate, which may lead to the development of dampness and decay. It is this very fact that has come to public notice in recent times. In Cleveland, Ohio, just a few years ago, a dramatic health problem arose among infants who lived in substandard accommodations. The common feature associated with these outbreaks was a fungal growth on the wet interior wallboards of the buildings. These microbes possessed powerful toxins that were present in their airborne spores. Scientists have suggested that when these spores were inhaled, the toxins inhaled with them led to the development of dramatic respiratory malfunction, which sometimes resulted in death.[283] Such episodes remind us of related observations made many years previously when fungal growth on damp wallpaper released toxic arsenic gases. Not surprisingly, these gases adversely affected people inhaling them.[284] Today, there is considerable public interest in "sick building syndrome" and "building related illness." Some of the episodes may be associated with building dampness and the growth of microbes. The effects of such microbial activity are apparently able to adversely influence human health, causing problems to the immune, neurological, and respiratory systems and the skin.[285]

Highlight: *Human activities lead to degradation of soil, air, water, and space. Understanding the nature of these impacts helps us to consider how we can make a difference and live more intelligently and healthfully.*

In the following section, I deal briefly with some of the motivating thoughts that energize people to care for the environment.

Care of the Natural World

As already indicated in our introduction, cities are places where pollution is most likely to be experienced. Such pollution impacts people's health and may lead to acute and chronic respiratory diseases.[286] We must not imagine that the ancient cities had no experiences of pollution. Human and animal waste disposal have always been problems in cities and some, like selected ancient Roman cities, had very advanced systems to dispose of waste, as illustrated in the ruins at Ephesus, Turkey. Civilizations before and after have been plagued by pollution of the environment.

In order to illustrate, we might mention that early Arabic treatises (as early as the ninth and tenth centuries) spoke about air and water pollution and their effect on human health.[287] Later, King Edward 1 of England banned the use of sea-coal in 1272 in order to improve air quality in London. This had little practical impact because supplies of coal were plentiful and the alternative (wood) was expensive. Real progress only commenced after 1952 when mass deaths occurred as a result of air pollution. Often progress has had priority over other concerns, as in the case seen in England over hundreds of years.[288] The same attitude prevails today in many countries irrespective of the philosophy adopted.

> *If we destroy the environment we are really guilty of destroying evidence that is meant to lead us to understand the ways of the Creator of the universe.*

There is an interesting comment recorded by the Christian prophet known as John the revelator who wrote in the first century of the present era. He made the dramatic statement that the God in whom he trusted would return one day and, among other things, would "destroy those who destroy the earth" (Revelation 11:18). Part of the reason for this rebuke evidently was that the "book of nature" has not been appreciated. It has been placed at our disposal for our enjoyment and to aid in our understanding of God's character and to lead others to recognize that He is the author of the laws of nature (Romans 1:20; 2:14, 15). In other words, the writer is saying that if we destroy the environment we are really guilty of destroying evidence that is meant to lead us to understand the ways of the Creator of the universe. The moral flaws in humans run very deep. The graphic statements of the prophet Hosea (4:1–10) link moral departures with ecological disaster. Is it too great a step to suggest that the same pattern is happening today?

If we follow the reasoning of proto-Christian writers, we find that the creator God placed the original human pair in a garden setting watered by magnificent rivers (Genesis 2:8–10). This place was not subjected to death and pollution, for intense agricultural and husbandry activities did not commence until after the initial human pair disobeyed the specific instruction given to them by their benefactor (Genesis 3:17–19). The original pair was given a caretaker role of the Garden of Eden and the environment (Genesis 2:15). Moreover, they were to "fill the earth" (Genesis 1:28), but not overfill it.

When Jesus lived in the land of Palestine (about two thousand years ago), He chose country locations for His greatest evangelistic endeavors and frequently took illustrations from nature to emphasize spiritual lessons. He chose country settings for rest and reflection with His disciples rather than lodging at a crowded resort (Mark 6:31), thus He indicated His preference for simplicity where possible and His interest in nature.

Highlight: The care of nature is part of the responsibility that must be recognized by those accepting the Christian tradition.

In the following section, I look at several examples of advanced practices used by some ancient cultures that impacted positively on the environment and I will derive some principles from the Scriptures on care of the environment.

Environmental Care and Planning for Healthy Living

Communities of animals, plants, and other living organisms form part of an ecosystem and interact in complex ways that ensures the continuance of community members. The complexity of the interactions found in such systems ensures that slight to moderate perturbations will be rectified and the system will return to its basal state. The terrestrial ecosystem includes humans as community members. Disruption of the ecosystem occurs when habitat destruction is widespread and non-selective, when pollution is mindlessly and continually practiced, and fire, flood, changes in temperature, migration of species, and other phenomena are impacting on the environment in uncharacteristic frequency.

Human population increase and greed are root causes of many environmental issues experienced today. It is assumed by some that this filling of the earth by humanity was to be endless, yet others disagree. I side with those who find that endless filling was not part of the ongoing instruction to humanity (cf. new earth population dynamics—Matthew 22:30 and the mandate of survival of all saved species taught by the flood episode—Genesis 7:1–3). The instruction to multiply and fill the earth must not be seen as an excuse to reduce biodiversity through habitat destruction. The food given to humans in the beginning was also to sustain the animals (Genesis 1:29, 30), and God's covenant after the flood included all living things, not only human beings (Genesis 9:10–12). Thus, we should be mindful of God's wishes and not frustrate His purpose.[289]

One can read into the instruction given by God to build the ark that earth's resources could be used to satisfy the necessities for human survival needs, but that the fate of the animal population (basal kinds created) was vitally important and was in human hands under stewardship arrangements (Genesis 6:14–22). Furthermore, the Scriptures later inform us that all creation seeks deliverance and that an account will be required of the responsibility displayed by humanity (Romans 8:20–23; Colossians 1:16; Revelation 11:18).[290] I suggest that this understanding also is resident in the fuller concept of the Sabbath rest, which included rest for livestock in the beginning.[291] We should not be found destroying evidences of God's character seen in His second book of information—nature.[292] I will comment on the conservation principles that can be derived from Scripture shortly.

There are other concepts upheld in the Bible designed to maintain the health and happiness of God's creation. These principles encompass first the physical, mental, social and spiritual dimensions of human health. In the context of this book, the spiritual dimension is paramount as pointed out by King Solomon as follows: "Trust in the Lord with all your heart … in all your ways acknowledge Him … fear the Lord…. It will be health to your flesh and strength to your bones" (Proverbs 3:5–8). The nub of the argument put by Solomon is that those who acknowledge God's claims and seek an understanding of His ways and commit to right doing will find peace and health (Proverbs 3:1–35; cf. Psalm 37:1–8). There is a wealth of information in the action words "acknowledging," "fearing," and "keeping" God's moral principles and guidelines. I would argue that realization of the principles of human health and their adoption by Christians ultimately will lead to a desire to improve ecosystem health, for the clear thinking individual understands that nature informs us of the character of God (Romans 1:20).

Highlight: The earth is under stewardship arrangements from God. This places a solemn responsibility on humans to act to bring glory to God and care for His creation.

Some ancient cultural practices have little modern relevance, but others were advanced in their logic and scientific soundness, although we are not claiming that the reasons for success were clearly understood by individuals living many centuries ago. A number of fundamental principles can be established from Scripture in relation to ecosystem community health that may be summarized under three headings.

Genetic Diversity

> *The first conservation principle...is the need to maintain genetic diversity so that unrepresentative characteristics do not arise.*

It must be admitted by all that the genetic resources preserved by the people surviving the great flood were much less than those available in the entire population destroyed (the same applies to all the animal groups taken into the ark). This meant that the post-Flood population was at risk for the simple reason that a lot of interbreeding with close relatives was bound to take place. Such populations tend to develop distinct characteristics, which differ from that observed in the original population. The first conservation principle that I

wish to highlight is the need to maintain genetic diversity so that unrepresentative characteristics do not arise. Recognition of this principle requires a little background.

There is suggestive evidence that over a period of approximately 500 years in early human history, after the great flood, that significant changes began to occur in the longevity of the human population (Genesis 9:28, 29; 11:10–26) causing God to instruct the race that inbreeding among closely related humans now was a restricted activity (cf. Genesis 12:13; Leviticus 18:6–14).[293] Perhaps the lack of fidelity to the original genome pattern was part of the reason for this instruction. In other words, operational deficiencies began to develop among the human population and reasonable changes needed to be introduced in breeding arrangements.

Some of the lifespan changes may have been due to mutations, as commonly observed today in experimental animals, and this may have led to a corresponding loss of longevity in humans. Indeed, it is generally conceded that many small mutations contribute to lifespan changes,[294] although there are some rare mutations that have considerable negative impacts on lifespan.[295] Another clue to the loss of longevity may be found in considering the close inbreeding that occurred after the flood in conjunction with possible genetic defects arising. To all intents and purposes the immediate post-flood population was isolated and the genetic diversity that they displayed was restricted, for they represented a closely related family unit, at least on the male side.[296] Furthermore, they were forced to engage in inbreeding activity to ensure succeeding generations arose. This raises the real possibility that if this population already possessed or indeed developed a mutational defect, then the effects of the deficiency would have been amplified. This idea of defect amplification arising in populations coming from a small number of individuals is amply supported by studies such as those involving the Ashkenazi Jews (primarily German Jews), the Amish, and the Newfoundland population.[297] An early founder population identified was the Jews of the Babylonian captivity of the sixth century before Christ. An X-linked disorder (important in red blood cell metabolism) that was present among them was accentuated by restrictions on intermarriage with non-Hebrews. Along similar lines, the continued ethnic isolation in Kurdistan Jews has led to an increased frequency of the deficiency in this group as opposed to the Yemen Jews who married more widely.[298]

Differences in the susceptibility of human populations and individuals to disease may be contributed to by genetic differences.[299] From animal studies, it is known that restricting the robustness of the genetic pool in animals (such as in founder and in endangered populations) may lead to greater risks of the population being eliminated through infection, as I will document presently. Similar outcomes may have been experienced among human population groups.

Genetic diversity can be altered through the continual presence of disease. This phenomenon has been observed in animal and human populations in response to selected diseases.[300] Sometimes the interactions between host and pathogen lead to the emergence of milder strains of the disease organism and more resistant hosts. At other times, changes are noted in the host that may lead to deleterious effects on physical performance. More worrying are instances, where through restricted out breeding and other factors, a more susceptible population to disease has emerged.[301] This means that it is possible that restriction in the robustness of the genetic pool in animals (such as seen in founder and endangered populations) may lead to greater risks of the population being eliminated through infection. Indeed, this has been found with captive cheetahs where a high proportion of the population may be susceptible to virus disease and elimination.[302] More interestingly the

rats on Christmas Island were rendered extinct by an introduced protozoan parasite, and the Tasmanian devil population currently is endangered by disease.[303] Similarly, in agricultural crops, planting large areas to a single genotype invites disaster from disease agents and weeds. Using a number of plant genotypes, varying the crops grown, and changing management practices all contribute toward reducing losses.[304]

Highlight: The first conservation principle that we can enunciate is that genetic diversity must be maintained at all costs for higher forms of life by preserving populations of animals (including humans) and plants in the various locations in the world where they occur.

Preserving and Repairing the Environment

The apostle Paul, under inspiration, reminds us that "we know that the whole creation groans and labors with birth pangs together until now" (Romans 8:22). And the psalmist tells us that heaven and earth "will all grow old like a garment" (Psalm 102:26). In Isaiah 24 we have a prophetic vision of the consequences of human folly in the earth (verses 3–12). The earth lies polluted under its inhabitants because "they have broken the laws, disobeyed the statutes and violated the eternal covenant" (verse 5, NEB). The prophet goes on to describe the utter destruction of the world (verses 19, 20). This could mean that God's judgments will destroy the earth and its inhabitants or that the human race through its activities, under the guidance of Satan, will bring about their own destruction (and God will not intervene to prevent the destruction of humanity). The rejection of the everlasting covenant by humans is seen in the disregard of the provision God has made for their salvation. In their supposed wisdom, humans have presumed to find alternative explanations for origins and routes to a better life. They often are not interested in the restoration of the image of God in humanity (Genesis 3:15; Romans 9:21–23; Revelation 14:6, 7).

Humans are still a steward of God's creation despite the entrance of sin (Psalm 8:6). Christ's sacrifice has enlightened our minds, sensitized them to the suffering of all creation, and given us responsibility to alleviate this misery (Romans 8:22; 2 Corinthians 4:3–6; Revelation 11:18). The delicate structure of the natural world and the value of its preservation and study are recognized in Scripture,[305] and a clear conservation principle is established through the great flood experience—all God's creatures are valuable in His sight (Genesis 7:1–3, 23). A specific statement regarding the necessity for conservation is given in Deuteronomy 22:6, 7. Here it is forbidden to snare and kill a female (bird) and her young. The breeding stock was to be preserved although the young could be taken. This again indicates to us that God is interested in the survival of His creatures (cf. Luke 12:6). The well-being of domestic creatures is also considered in the scriptural record. They were provided for in the Sabbath rest instructions and at other times the needs of beasts that served humanity were sensitively provided (Deuteronomy 5:14, 15; 25:4).

The Scriptures clearly recognize the need to act wisely to control wild animals, which may have increased to the point where they endangered agriculture and life itself (Exodus 23:29; Leviticus 26:6). Such activities were to be done humanely, for we learn a principle of action in Proverbs 12:10 (NEB). It says, "A righteous man cares for his beast, but a wicked man is cruel at heart." The ancient children of God were committed to the conservation of the productivity of agricultural lands and to the maintenance of tree resources. They practised a period of rest of agricultural lands every seventh year (Exodus 23:11; Leviticus 25:1–7), which served to control diseases and increase productivity in the initial years of the next cycle. The practice also impressed upon them

continually that they were not to exhaust the land. Resources were to be valued and used judiciously. Their concern for fruit tree resources is shown by the strict instructions given to conquering armies. They were not to destroy them, "for the tree of the field is man's food" (Deuteronomy 20:19). The practices adopted by the Israelites were in contrast to those of contemporary cultures where the custom was to destroy gardens and useful trees.[306]

The children of Israel were also taught to value natural resources, and they were not to view them as inexhaustible. This is clearly illustrated by reference to Isaiah 9:9–11 (NEB), where the Lord in His anger with the Jews threatened to destroy them because, among other things, "in their pride and arrogance they say, the bricks are fallen, but we will build in hewn stone; the sycamores are hacked down, but we will use cedars instead." We can gain a brief glimpse of God's attitude toward restoration of the environment from Ezekiel 47. If His representatives had followed His principles lush pastures, forests, and teeming multitudes of animals would have replaced deserts and sparsely populated regions at His command (verses 2–10).

In seeking to restore the environment and protect various life forms a difficult question is: What exactly are we seeking to protect and restore? The life forms we have with us today are not the originals. Indeed, some forms may have been changed remarkably by both human manipulation and by satanic agencies. Perhaps we might suggest that priorities be given to those activities that are devoted to preserving/restoring beauty (Luke 12:27), promoting helpful/cooperative elements (Genesis 7:2),[307] and assisting the establishment of harmonious relationships (Isaiah 65:25; cf. Genesis 7:2; Leviticus 11:2–23). In making these statements, I certainly acknowledge the value of protecting the total gene pool available if possible, for valuable genes conferring resistance to disease or ability to survive tough environments may be found there. In addition, some seemingly unprofitable organisms may prove to be of considerable value in the future.[308]

Few areas of the world retain an ecosystem in a pristine condition. Where such are present, they should be preserved in order to maintain genetic diversity on the one hand and to give additional examples to humanity of the handiwork of God—His second book of information is to be preserved! Indeed, the Sabbath links the creation event to acknowledgment by humans of being made in the image of God, and it continues to instruct us to preserve His second book of information—nature.[309]

Highlight: The second conservation principle that we can enunciate is that conserving and repairing the environment is a responsibility of every Christian, for it represents an essential part of preserving God's second book of information—nature—and bringing honor to Him.

Health Awareness and Predisposition to Disease

Health in humans is vital for the preservation of God's creation, for it leads to clear thinking. Maintaining the marvellous machinery in peak condition brings glory to God (1 Corinthians 10:31). It is the purpose of this book to outline the Bible principles of health involved. Now these have implications for both the animal and plant populations. For animals, both balanced nutrition and social health are vital to their proper functioning and to assist in protecting them from disease. For plants, balanced nutrition is essential to give them the best advantages in resisting disease. It is considered that supplying all the known nutrients in balance stimulates optimal growth and this generally ensures superior disease resistance.[310]

A holistic approach to health brings the responsibilities of the human instrument into focus concerning their ambassadorial role.

A holistic approach to health brings the responsibilities of the human instrument into focus concerning their ambassadorial role (2 Corinthians 5:20) and response to God's generous offer of salvation (Hebrews 2:3). Our responsibilities to care for God's creation become clearer as we accept God's salvation makeover (2 Corinthians 3:18; 4:6) and understand that God's redemptive act was to rescue all of creation (Romans 8:19–21). This is again clearly evident in the Sabbath rest, which is meant to embrace not only humans but domestic animals too (Exodus 20:10; 23:12).

Highlight: The third conservation principle that we can enunciate is that the maintenance of good health maximizes the possibilities of avoiding disease in animals (including human) and plants and assists in their survival and optimal functioning.

There are two examples of practices mentioned in the Bible that are relevant to maintaining a healthy living environment that I will mention in greater detail in the chapter on protection. The association between careful human waste disposal and freedom from disease was understood when the Israelite slaves escaped from Egyptian captivity (around 1447 BC).[311] They were advised to bury fecal material to ensure that public health was maintained (Deuteronomy 23:12, 13); this is in marked contrast to the medical practices in Egypt at the time where human and animal excrement was used frequently to treat disease.[312]

One very perceptive piece of advice taught in the same tradition (Jewish) related to the condition of permanent dwellings (Leviticus 14:37–45). A common practice around the mid-fifteenth century before the present era was that if a dwelling showed signs of mildew (growth of microbes) or perhaps dry rot (fungal growth) then something dramatic needed to be done by the homeowner under instruction from those in authority.[313] The advice was that replacement and repair should be tried first, but if this failed the building was to be destroyed. This is entirely sound and responsible bearing in mind economic and health issues. Dry rot compromises structural integrity while damp induces growth of microbes that can have serious health outcomes, as we have noted already from our example taken from Cleveland, Ohio. We recorded previously that fungal growth on the wet wall boards of buildings in Cleveland was associated provisionally with the death of some infants through the inhalation of toxins produced by the molds. Living and work environments are something that many cannot change radically, but being informed is the first step toward doing what is in our power to change.

Highlight: *Selected practices from ancient Jewish literature indicates that their ideas on the disposal of fecal waste and on the care of residential buildings were sound to a remarkable degree giving renewed interest in these scriptures.*

Some Cultural Advice on Community Living

In the last section in this chapter, I will deal briefly with advice on community living. Today most of us find ourselves living under crowded conditions in cities, ostensibly giving greater opportunity to become involved in community affairs. However, the sobering fact is that, in our day, people in industrialized societies are becoming less community orientated and have focused on success and self-interest rather than on group interests.[314] A careful look at communities shows that society is more the focus of attention where Eastern-based philosophies prevail while Western philosophy has induced people to focus more on the individual.[315]

In Western societies another phenomenon has become evident. Many are reacting against appeals to reason that have characterized modern life. The rational approach has been responsible for the advances gained through science and the discovery of the laws of nature that are used for the benefit of humanity. Those who reject a reasoned approach blame the problems of our time on the scientific approach and choose rather to be directed by their emotions.[316] Such individuals may be found in the endless pursuit of pleasure. Life for them becomes a carnival where all convention is left behind and the reveler sets to enjoying all the novel experiences that may be imagined.[317]

Now the adverse influence of some modern developments in science on society and the environment sometimes have been attributed to Christian attitudes, particularly those relating to humans being seen as separate and superior to nature.[318] While this is not the place to analyze this thesis, one can say that the human race alone was created in God's image and was left in charge of other forms of life (Genesis 1:27, 28). Indeed, some of the attitudes expressed by Christians make them poor ambassadors for their faith both in terms of community responsibility and the related issue of environmental care.

In order to highlight this linkage, we might remind readers that those who practice love toward their neighbors do not wantonly use resources to selfishly serve their needs with no consideration being given either to present populations in other areas of the world or to future populations, including their own offspring. A model of sustainability and responsibility is an overdue response by informed Christians.[319]

There is a balance of thoughts found within the Christian philosophy regarding community living and environmental responsibility. This is perhaps not surprising, as this philosophy arose in the East. The advice by one of its most profound biblical scholars (Paul) is that "let us consider one another in order to stir up love and good works" (Hebrews 10:24). The principal source of information on relationships in the Christian tradition is considered to have come from God, the Creator of the human race. He directed people to consider His basic instruction uncluttered by human speculations and declarations (Matthew 15:1–3; 19:3–10). In fact, one of the dramatic effects of the human race disobeying their Creator was that soon after the commencement of the colonization of planet earth individual concerns displaced community concerns (Genesis 3:2–13; cf. Genesis 2:23, 24). An attempt to reverse this tendency was made by Christ's early disciples who lived by God's principles. They attempted to live together in unity, caring for each other (Acts 2:1, 44–47). They adopted the idea that community was given second place only in circumstances where higher principles could be identified (Acts 4:19, 20; 5:28, 29).

The concept of community is linked to the idea of ultimate purpose for the human race in the minds of some thinkers.

The concept of community is linked to the idea of ultimate purpose for the human race in the minds of some thinkers. Such individuals find this linkage of ideas flows freely from the concept that life arose by means other than pure chance. If we live among and/or observe nature, we are impressed with the very complexity that we see in the world about us, particularly in the intricate biochemistry of the simplest organism. It is not surprising that this causes many to view the emergence of life forms arising through random events as having an exceedingly small possibility of success.

Intelligent involvement in the design of nature is something that many agree comes logically from the massed evidence accumulated by the various sciences. For example, even the simplest organism needs complex processes in order to operate, and multiple processes are needed for the operation of its many cellular systems. This means that even the simplest free-living organisms known are both intricate in design and have many interlinking processes necessary for integrity and multiplication. This complexity cannot be reduced while still retaining cell function.[320] If this concept appears hard to grasp, just try to simplify an uncomplicated mechanical device and still retain its function. The vital question is: How could such complexity as observed in cells arise step by step? Like the philosophers the apostle Paul interacted with in the early years of the present era (Romans 1: 21), many modern thinkers have no need for God because they prefer to glory in human imagination. They attempt to eliminate problems about beginnings and laws of the universe through appeals to random events and vast periods of time. This simply represents a device to transfer the problem, not to solve it. They need faith to support their intellectual enterprise.

The challenge given to all earth's inhabitants by the Christian scriptures is that the Supreme God highlighted in its pages plans to create a new world free from the rule by fang, tooth, and selfishness (Isaiah 65:17–25, Revelation 21:1–5). This poses a remarkable problem for those who believe that this world was created by God through the process of evolution. The nature of the problem is stated rather forcefully some years ago in the premier scientific journal *Nature* under the title: "The God of the Galápagos." It was argued that a god who commenced the creation process and then allowed the face of nature to change under the rule of fang and claw (survival of the fittest) "is not the Protestant God of waste not, want not. He is also not a loving God who cares about His productions. He is not even the awful god portrayed in the book of Job. The God of the Galápagos is careless, wasteful, indifferent, almost diabolical. He is certainly not the sort of God to whom anyone would be inclined to pray."[321] This perception contrasts rather poorly with the claim that God is a loving and compassionate God and worthy of worship. Will such a God save us? The answer is that "No, such a god is incapable of saving anyone." Such a God is not the God of those who believe implicitly in the Holy Bible.

The God of Bible-loving Christians shows us that care for human communities and the environment arise from the concept of God's love (*agape* type). This is the love that reached down to save humanity by suffering an ignominious death on the cross, this is the love that will create a new heavens and earth, this is the love that presents a consistent picture of communion and concern for rebellious humanity and appeals to all hearers and readers. The love was expressed by Jesus Christ and is ours to accept by faith and rejoice in.

Highlight: *Community involvement is valued by Eastern cultures and philosophies and this includes Christianity, which arose in the East. Recapturing the spirit of community involvement and interest will make the world in which we live a richer place and contribute to more rewarding and healthful living.*

Guiding Principles and Practical Suggestions

1. Soil degradation may lead to plant deficiencies. Among the human population, it has been found that eating extensively of plant varieties able to more efficiently extract nutrients from soils reduces the chances of deficiency diseases developing.

2. Soil pollution may occur as a result of waste from industries being deposited or polluted water being used.

3. Soil nutrients are lost by erosion. Water erosion may be prevented by restricted land clearing, especially near watercourses, by the planting of trees in depressions where drainage water runs or by terracing hillsides (or contouring bank construction). Wind erosion may be minimized by maintaining effective plant cover of soil, by planting tree or shrub wind brakes, constructing artificial wind brakes, or covering the soil with organic waste or crop residues.

4. Produce taken off the land effectively reduces the supply of nutrient reserves present in the soil. The plant nutrients generally requiring attention are nitrogen, phosphorus, and potassium. Crop rotations involving legumes may effectively add nitrogen and humus if the green legume crop is returned to the soil. Other nutrients, when depleted, must be added from an outside source.

5. Water quality loss means a loss of livelihood, habitat, beauty, and the ability to enjoy restful activities in a particular locale. The more insidious effects are increases in disease producing chemical agents in water systems, which give rise to changes in the animals still living there. Toxic chemicals have been found in the fish in polluted areas and toxins may exceed levels considered fit for human consumption.

6. Water quality loss is everyone's responsibility. Rubbish and industrial wastes, when discarded indiscriminately, will inevitably

find their way into watercourses and pollute. Excess nutrients, such as industrial wastes, fertilizer run-off, and sewage, destroy water quality. Judicious use of fertilizers and the planting of protective strips of grasses and trees adjacent to watercourses can limit nutrient pollution.

7. Growing food crops on areas contaminated with heavy metals and taking seafoods from waters contaminated by industrial and sewage is a poor option.

8. The poor quality of city air has long been known to cause health problems such as acute and chronic respiratory diseases. Dampness and decay associated with buildings may influence human health. Improving air quality is a community responsibility in which the ordinary citizen may participate. This may involve adding one's voice of concern to the political debate, participating in community pollution minimization schemes, using public transport, carpooling, maintaining vehicles properly, and reducing the use of fossil fuels.

9. Damp proofing buildings or choosing dry building sites will aid in the minimization of some respiratory diseases associated with microbes. Proper maintenance and cleaning of air conditioning systems also assists in keeping good air quality standards and avoiding disease.

10. Breathing air contaminated by particles of matter (inorganic or organic) is not conducive to health whether they are organic or inorganic.

11. City living encourages crime and the pursuit of pleasure seeking activities.

12. Population pressures lead to various adverse outcomes. Among these it is found that small living spaces influence the feeling of well-being and change human behavior; children's imagination is limited.

13. Crowding in the zones outside the living quarters also affects one's sense of well-being, leading to a sense of disorientation or oppression, loss of a caring attitude, and frustration.

14. In a crowd, the rational faculties of the individual are lowered so that a crowd mentality is established. Some suggest that individuals immersed in a crowd event behave like individuals under hypnosis.

15. Nature is ours to enjoy and respect. Destroying it wantonly raises questions of moral responsibility.

16. Conservation principles established from a biblical base indicate that God made a covenant to preserve all created species, in these genetic diversity should be maintained, and the health of living things maintained to the best of our ability.

17. If preservation priorities have to be made, then some preference might be given to project that preserve and restore beauty, promote helpful and cooperative relationships, and assist the development of harmonious relationships.

18. Our responsibility is to God, society, and our families. Community values and responsibilities need to be emphasized in societies, for no individual or nation can live in isolation. It represents a shallow morality if we ignore community responsibilities and the fate of God's second book of information—nature.

Chapter 6

Protection

Preventive medicine is a relatively recent concept. Diseases have long afflicted the human race. Their cause and cure was debated by the ancients, and some novel and challenging cures were suggested. Hippocrates (the father of medicine) and Galen were two famous physicians of antiquity who wrote and taught on these subjects. They focused on describing diseases and suggesting how they might be cured. Besides these students of natural science, Hindu and Chinese sages and healers in other cultures devised their own strategies for curing disease.[322]

The modern era was late in adopting practices that could prevent the development of disease. The cause of many common diseases to afflict humanity has been solved within a little over the last 100 years. Some individuals stand particularly tall in our memories for advancing knowledge of disease and how to prevent it. They all taught contrary to popular belief. We will mention just four of these people—Robert Koch, Joseph Lister, Louis Pasteur, and Ignaz Semmelweis, although this does some injustice to others.

Koch is remembered to this day for his discovery of the bacterium that causes the highly infectious disease known as anthrax. He nominated a series of steps, still practiced, to establish a causal relationship between an organism and disease. Pasteur is remembered among other things for work supporting the germ theory of disease, the development of vaccines, and for the pasteurization process used in wine and dairy products, which we use today to kill dangerous microbes potentially found in many food items. Before these scientists made their momentous discoveries, the Austrian physician Semmelweis had noticed that washing the hands in antiseptic after performing an autopsy substantially reduced deaths in women in childbirth. Now, strange as it sounds, doctors generally did not bother to carry out any sanitary processes, such as washing their hands, before attending the women. Although Semmelweis's work was generally ridiculed, Joseph Lister in England accepted the advances made by Louis and Semmelweis and went on to pioneer the use of antiseptics in surgery.[323] The results were very satisfying, and it is hardly possible to conceive of life without the use of such procedures.

Before these modern advances, it may surprise readers to learn that the Old Testament prophet Moses gave some sound instructions, under God's direction, that would have gone a long way toward preventing a number of significant diseases. We will briefly review these, but in doing so I am not suggesting that Moses or those who came after him understood why the procedures adopted worked. It also is important for readers to note that in today's world some of the practices highlighted have been superseded by more modern procedures, which accomplish similar disease escape or control outcomes.

Contagious Nature of Some Diseases

We well remember the lepers who stood a long way from Jesus and cried out: "Jesus, Master, have mercy on us!" (Luke 17:13). By the laws of society, these unfortunate people had to be isolated and to advertise their condition by crying "Unclean! Unclean!" (Leviticus 13:45, 46). This essentially said that the disease was infectious and could be transmitted to others through contact. Furthermore, it suggested that human beings could be a reservoir of the disease.

Now if we think about the biblical laws governing disease outbreaks in general among individuals and the precautions suggested for handling contaminated clothing and articles and how to deal with ugly discoloured patches in damp houses (Leviticus 11, 13–15), the inevitable conclusion must be reached that a variety of illnesses and diseases and conditions could be minimized or prevented by adopting sensible precautions. I will take some examples to illustrate this.

Disease may be transmitted by contact with an infected individual as well as with soiled articles of clothing and bedding. The instruction given to those contaminated with body discharges coming from an unwell person was to wash both their body and clothes and the infected individual was to do likewise when they had recovered (Leviticus 15:3–13). Here we have an indication that both direct and indirect transmission of infection could take place. The simple exercise of washing would effectively minimize the risk of cross infection occurring. The soundness of this advice is seen when considering some food-poisoning organisms that primarily are transmitted via the fecal-oral route. By this we mean that organisms carried in waste material can contaminate the hands and may then move readily to food items and hence back into the body.

Modern science has shown that even the simple act of washing the hands in water will reduce the possibility of effective transfer taking place; the effect is strengthened by using various soaps.[324] The biblical instruction given to those contaminated with soiled material from sick people involved washing and then exposure to air and possibly sunlight, as the individuals were considered unclean until nightfall. This combination of procedures would have been much more effective in neutralizing dangerous organisms than the act of simply washing, as every modern microbiologist is aware.[325]

Highlight: Maintaining cleanliness of person after touching infected individuals, clothing, and bedding is a sound practice to adopt in attempts to minimize infection by disease causing organisms.

The biblical record remains unclear about the identity of some diseases described in its pages. Leprosy (Hansen's disease) was recognized in antiquity as well as schistosomiasis, malaria, smallpox, and tuberculosis. Of these, leprosy and tuberculosis are transmissible. However, we cannot be certain about the time of their appearance.[326]

One of the most spectacular examples of contaminated articles causing disease comes from considering the smallpox organism. This virus has now been eradicated from the world, but it appeared on the scene before 1000 BC as an endemic disease in Egypt. There is evidence of smallpox in mummies from the eighteenth and twentieth dynasties, and some believe it was present much earlier. There is uncertainty over the exact time these dynasties occurred, which makes application of God's promise to the Israelites to keep them free from dangerous diseases difficult to align with the exodus (1447 BC according to the new chronology). However, we know that the Hittite armies attacked Egypt in the fourteenth century BC, but were decimated by an infectious disease contracted from Egyptian captives. The devastation lasted for at least twenty years and claimed commoners and royalty alike. Some believe this epidemic was caused by smallpox.[327]

Smallpox may have arisen in central Africa well before the time of the exodus. Some read into ancient Egyptian documents dating as early as 3000 BC descriptions of a disease reminiscent of smallpox.[328] The history of its elimination and misuse illustrates our point about the mechanisms for spread of the disease. During natural infections, it was observed that those afflicted commonly had experienced close contact with victims. Hence, it is not surprising that during the eradication program contacts of infected individuals first were vaccinated and they were isolated if they showed

any signs of illness. This approach was very effective in all communities affected around the world. In hospital situations, contaminated bedding was disinfected according to strict protocols. These strategies led to the elimination of this dreaded disease. Unfortunately, an understanding of the infectious nature of this virus also allowed it to be used in a sinister manner—biological warfare. For example, during the French and Indian wars in North America (commenced 1754), the unscrupulous took blankets from smallpox sufferers and gave them to the Indians. The disease epidemics that followed were responsible for over half the tribal populations being eliminated.[329]

Transmission of leprosy is still something of an enigma. In most countries, humans appear to be the main source of the disease, although soil from the residential area of patients frequently contains the organism as can water found in endemic areas. On balance, it is considered that the organism enters primarily through contaminated droplets expelled from the nose and mouth of sufferers entering the body's respiratory system and through skin-to-skin contact.[330] This gives credibility to the biblical cautions about isolating those with the disease.

Highlight: *Diseases mentioned in Scripture have been identified with partial success and some infectious diseases were among these. The quarantine of individuals with these infectious diseases still is considered sound practice.*

Managing Human Waste and Contamination

The problem of separating ourselves from our waste products continues to be a significant challenge today irrespective of where we live. Lack of personal hygiene is highly significant in accounting for general health and for food safety issues. To illustrate, in one Middle East country, recent figures show that less than 30 percent of people clean their hands after toilet activities; not surprisingly problems arise in that foodborne infections are at an unsatisfactory high level.[331]

By contrast, this is not likely to happen to orthodox Jews. They are instructed to wash their hands before any holy act or prayer, before and after a meal, and after touching an unclean object or performing certain bodily functions (see also Leviticus 7:21). These practices have come from antiquity and contain both physical and ritual elements. The biblical basis for such customs comes from a number of texts (e.g., Exodus 30:19; Leviticus 15:11; Psalm 26:6), but also contain interpretive elements based on the idea that "cleanliness is next to godliness." The washing is done with pure water.[332] Today modern societies accept the interpretative elements as scientific truth. The ritual elements emphasized the holiness of God (source of life) in contrast to states/activities that pointed to death, decay, and wasted life forces.

The disposal of human waste was given particular attention by Moses.

The disposal of human waste was given particular attention by Moses, as briefly mentioned already. As they journeyed the Israelites were to be careful to bury solid human waste (Deuteronomy 23:12–14). This served a number of functions. First, the fly population was prevented from carrying microbes from this waste material to the eyes and mouths of the young, and movement of microbes from human feces to food was prevented. A reasonable number of foodborne illnesses and eye and other diseases are associated with the activities of the domestic fly. They have been implicated in other serious diseases such

as tuberculosis, cholera and typhoid fever, and a number of illnesses caused by viruses.[333]

Secondly, the burden of disease coming from parasitic worms was reduced. Today, it is known that poor sanitation (and also using untreated fecal material in agriculture) and contaminated water promote worm infections in poor societies. Even today, high burdens of specialized worms are found in East Asia. Their life cycles center on escape from the body via the feces. They contaminate the environment and commonly re-enter the body through the skin or intestinal tract (some may be transmitted by insects).[334]

The third benefit of burying human waste was to reduce the possibility of contamination of water sources. The provision of safe water is one of the prime requirements for the maintenance of health. Contamination by microbes arising from fecal matter causes diarrheal disease (cholera, typhoid, viruses). Disease may then be transferred person-to-person, if hand washing and other hygienic practices are not adopted.[335] Aid agencies understand this linkage well and make strenuous efforts to provide safe sanitary disposal facilities for waste and clean water.

No comprehensive direct instruction is given in Scripture about keeping water sources clean, although limited advice is given about contamination of water by carcasses (Leviticus 11:35, 36). This advice was to ensure contamination of water did not occur beyond a minimal level. In addition, as noted above, Jews used pure water for hand washing rather than discoloured or contaminated sources. They were no doubt aware of the dire results that could arise from using contaminated water. For example, in ancient times all sorts of devices were used to disable enemies, which included poisoning their water supplies with plants and dead animals. Even during the American Civil War (1863) and the Kosovo conflict (1998), wells and other bodies of water were polluted with dead animals.[336]

Highlight: Sound management of human waste and avoiding contamination of water sources helps to reduce the level of disease found in communities.

Contamination of water, food, and hands with fecal matter often is responsible for the spread of a number of gastrointestinal diseases. All types of domesticated and wild animals and humans potentially are responsible for providing polluting materials and a considerable range of foods may be involved.[337] The involvement of fecal contamination has been demonstrated on a regular basis by the outbreak of disease following contamination of food and water supplies. For example, the pollution of an non-chlorinated water supply by elk and deer feces is thought to have been responsible for a large outbreak of gastrointestinal disease in Alpine, Wyoming, just a few years ago.[338] A variety of diseases may be traced to food and water containing fecal materials, irrespective of whether the country is poor or wealthy. It is a sad fact, however, that gastrointestinal diseases are responsible for a high rate of infant deaths in poor countries (up to seventeen fold differences have been noted between these countries and wealthy ones). The main factors responsible are access to sanitation and clean water.[339]

Protection Against Foodborne Diseases

The Hebrew people did not live in a scientific age, yet some sound advice was given to them regarding the keeping and eating of meat, which is very prone to decay, particularly in hot climates. In a brief account of practices associated with eating a portion of the peace offerings (cattle, sheep, goats—Numbers 7:17), no item was to be eaten beyond the second day (Leviticus 19:5, 6). The peace offerings were of ritual significance, expressing joy and fellowship with God[340]; nevertheless, the advice on time limits for keeping the food item

is sound, for the organisms carried on the meat following slaughter multiply rapidly.

The soundness of the advice can be illustrated by referring to other hot environments in the tropics (e.g., India). There it is usual for retailers to sell sheep carcasses held without refrigeration within eighteen to twenty hours. Off-odours become evident by the second or third day.[341]

Highlight: Food spoilage is one factor contributing to negative health outcomes.

Protection Against Sexually Transmitted Disease

The biblical instructions regarding protection against sexually transmitted diseases are not stated in scientific terms, but rather as moral guidelines. These, if followed, provide protection against sexually transmitted disease, whatever society is being spoken about. They are so clear that there should be no confusion, although some would argue that times have changed. This is as far from the truth as the east is from the west. God's standards do not change (Malachi 3:6). Christ gave His life to reconcile humans to God and to recreate the moral image of God in them (Romans 5:10; Colossians 1:20, 21)!

If we go back to the beginning, God created male and female to populate the earth (Genesis 1:27, 28; 2:18, 20–25). Furthermore, the Bible makes it clear that fidelity of the human family would be maintained by adhering to some rather simple and logical undertakings. By the time of Moses, these included prohibition of marriage to those closely related (see later), strict loyalty to the marriage arrangement, and no unusual relationships involving same sex or perversions involving animals (Exodus 20:14; Leviticus 18:20, 22–25). Unfortunately, the image of God in the human race was marred by the entrance of sin, and it continued to fade with time. A particularly powerful force in this decline was the perverted sexual relationships entered into (Leviticus 18:22–24; Romans 1:22–29; 1 Corinthians 5:1; Ephesians 5:3). These are rather graphically recorded in history, so there is no guesswork as to what the texts are referring to.[342]

The image of God in the human race was marred by the entrance of sin, and it continued to fade with time.

Jesus mentioned the very high standards expected of the human race (Matthew 5:27, 28), which included not only abstinence from sex before marriage but also purity of thought about the opposite sex. Hollywood and Bollywood fall far short in these areas and encourage others to enter into dangerous territory. So do believers in evolutionary theory. In one country surveyed (Australia) believers in Darwinism were found more permissible about pre-marital sex and abortion than those holding Christian beliefs, although not by a margin that would give cause for joy.[343]

Highlight: The moral image of God in humanity can be strengthened by respecting the sanctity of marriage and living in accordance with the code of sexual relationships outlined in Scripture.

Syphilis was encountered in some parts of the world an estimated 5,000 years ago. It came to prominence when Columbus's crew brought an aggressive form of the disease to the Old World some 500 years ago. It caused a sensation in Europe, being responsible for a destructive epidemic. There is no substantial evidence that it was found in Egypt at the time when the Israelites left for Canaan.[344] But no doubt other sexually transmitted diseases were found there.

Honouring the moral advice given in Scripture would lead to substantial decreases in syphilis and other sexually transmitted diseases. In order to illustrate, human immunodeficiency virus (HIV) infection suddenly appeared among those experimenting with sexual experiences outside those designed by God. All sorts of theories have been postulated as to the ultimate origin of the virus, which do not concern us here.[345] The appearance of the disease has led to untold tragedy with the innocent suffering along with those groups primarily responsible for the initial spread of the disease. These include those who do not have regard for the order established at creation, do not show marital fidelity, or who are intravenous drug users.[346]

Highlight: The incidence of sexually transmitted diseases is accentuated when practices are adopted outside those designed by God for the human race.

Protecting Populations

While we cannot treat the Bible as a scientific textbook, it does contain advice on community health.

There are certain characteristics shown or practices adopted by populations that predispose to disease. These include genetic background, general health (nutrition, overcrowding, and fatigue), immunization, age, gender, and religious and cultural practices.[347] While we cannot treat the Bible as a scientific textbook, it does contain advice on community health. Already we have dealt with predisposing elements such as nutrition, damp dwellings, and overcrowded environments on health. In the succeeding sections, I will give some insights into genetic background and cultural and religious practices. We will find that some of the principles established have not changed over time, whereas in other instances there are more modern equivalent practices that provide the same protective functions. Then again, novel solutions have been introduced, which have contributed enormously to advances in global health (e.g., antibiotics, immunization). Just as God gave sound advice anciently, He has provided the means to protect modern populations.

Genetic Diversity

In attempting to protect health, a significant principle that must be mentioned is the need to maintain genetic diversity and avoid a small number of individuals giving rise to a new population with limited genetic variability (founder effect). Recognition of this principle requires a little background. There is suggestive evidence that over a period of approximately 500 years in early human history significant changes began to occur in the human population, causing God to instruct the race that inbreeding among closely related humans was now a restricted activity (Genesis 12:13; Leviticus 18:6–14).[348]

Perhaps operational deficiencies began to develop among the human population so that reasonable changes needed to be introduced in the breeding arrangements given at creation. Some of the changes may have been due to mutations leading to a corresponding loss of longevity in humans. Indeed, it is generally conceded that many small mutations contribute to lifespan changes,[349] although there are some rare mutations that have considerable negative impacts on lifespan.[350] In selected experimental animals (mice), induction of premature aging may come through the introduction of mutational changes into a population. In this relatively recent experiment, it was found that when a vital enzyme was deleted premature death occurred (the mouse lifespan was reduced to about half). The mouse population also showed

baldness, osteoporosis, anemia, curvature of the spine, and reduced fertility.[351]

Support for the suggestion that the surviving population after or soon after the flood possessed or developed deficiencies comes from the biblical record. It says simply that whereas Noah lived 950 years (Genesis 9:29), the sons of Shem lived much shorter lives (Genesis 11:10–25). No doubt some of the children of Shem intermarried with the children of Ham and Japheth (Genesis 7:13), giving the possibility that the frequency of defects became more pronounced, leading to a progressive decline in the genetic robustness of the race. For those who are uncomfortable with God preserving a group of individuals carrying a genetic defect, it must be admitted by all that the genetic resources preserved by the people surviving the flood were much less than those available in the entire population destroyed (the same applies to all the animal groups taken into the ark). In addition, a defect arising soon after the flood event would have been amplified equally by the close interbreeding activities in the surviving community, thus leading to an overall similar result.

The genetic resources preserved by the people surviving the flood were much less than those available in the entire population destroyed.

Without dispute the immediate post-flood population was isolated and the genetic diversity that they displayed was restricted, for they represented a closely related family unit, at least on the male side.[352] Furthermore, they were forced to engage in intermarriage activity to ensure succeeding generations arose. This raises the real possibility that if this population already possessed or indeed developed a mutational defect, then the effects of the deficiency would have been amplified. The idea of defect amplification arising in populations coming from a founder group is amply supported by studies such as those involving the Ashkenazi Jews, the Amish, and the Newfoundland population.[353] An early founder population identified was the Jews of the Babylonian captivity of the sixth century before Christ. They possessed a disorder in red blood cell metabolism, and this was accentuated by restrictions on intermarriage with non-Hebrews. Along similar lines, the continued ethnic isolation in Kurdistan Jews has led to an increased frequency of the deficiency in this group as opposed to the Yemen Jews who married more widely.[354]

Highlight: Individuals surviving the universal flood were essentially a founder population and hence capable of accentuating genetic defects that might arise. These defects could have impacted negatively on general health and longevity.

We might be under the impression that marriage between close relatives is rare in today's world. This is a very mistaken idea. It is estimated that 8.4 percent of the world's children have related parents. In the West Asia, North Africa, and the Indian sub-continent at least 20–50 percent of marriages involve close relatives. Other communities (involving a billion people) look with favor on unions between second cousins or closer. It is no secret that neonatal and childhood death and disabilities are almost double in first cousin marriages.[355]

Highlight: Marriage between close relatives or when restricted to small communities has a greater risk of leading to the production of children with disabilities than when more options are considered for mate selection. Longevity issues may also be experienced when marriages are contracted between close relatives.

Perhaps another highly significant factor influencing lifespan expectations was the emergence of infectious microbial diseases. Disease tends to sweep away the genetically most susceptible members of the population. The first mention of infectious diseases was noted in the time of Job and again in the experiences of the children of Israel in Egypt (Deuteronomy 28:60; Job 2:7).[356] These would have allowed a variable proportion of the human population to have been eliminated at an early age. With some infectious diseases in the early stages of their introduction, it is possible that large numbers of individuals will be eliminated. Such a phenomenon was experienced during the conquest of the Americas, the black plague in Europe, the influenza epidemic of 1918, and is being experienced in the current HIV–AIDS epidemic.[357]

The genotype of the population would itself have been changed by the continual presence of disease, leading to genetic abnormalities and peculiarities. This scenario has been observed in animal and human populations in response to selected diseases.[358] For example, malaria has led to the emergence of a variety of genetic abnormalities among the human population[359] and the black plague has shaped the distribution of people suffering from iron overload.[360] All this selective pressure of disease and other factors has led to genetic differences being found in the susceptibility of human populations and individuals to disease.[361] Now restricting the robustness of the genetic pool in animals (such as in founder and in endangered populations) may lead to greater risks of the population being eliminated through infection.[362] Similar outcomes may have been experienced among human population groups.

Highlight: The selection pressure of diseases on the human population has led to the appearance of genetic differences. These may account partially for the variance in susceptibility of populations to disease.

Cultural and Religious Practices

In East London's crowded quarters at the turn the nineteenth century, health practitioners were fascinated to observe the lower rates of infant deaths among the Jewish population from infectious and respiratory diseases. This positive outcome has been explained by the close attention they gave to the biblical instructions on isolation and quarantine as well as to their interest in and attention to diet, the sparse use of alcohol, and personal hygiene. Personal hygiene requirements included hand washing before and after meals and keeping the surroundings clean. Utensils used in food preparation were also kept clean, and milk and meat were not mixed nor were the implements/utensils used to handle these food items.[363]

Besides these explanations, the escape from other diseases by the Jews during this period (e.g., cholera) has been attributed to the kosher preparation requirements for meat (resulted in there being fewer risks of diseased food being eaten), the practice of boiling water and milk, and using clean cooking and eating utensils. The religious laws also improved personal hygiene over the general population in that they required that nails be trimmed once a week and that women take a ritual bath once per month after menstruating. The immigrant Jews in London also customarily bathed on account of their general attitude toward cleanliness.[364]

Highlight: *Attention to personal hygiene, cleanliness of surroundings, and the use of food from sources less prone to microbial contamination contribute to the maintenance of good health.*

Looking at other practices, some religious groups have a strong tradition of male circumcision, a practice mentioned favorably in Scrip-

ture, but not imposed on the Christian church (Acts 7:8; 15:5, 28. 29). An interesting observation is that in those societies where the practice is accepted, there is an association with lower rates of cervical cancer and other sexually transmitted infections, including HIV. In a recent extensive analysis of trends across many countries in the developing world, the reduced incidence of HIV was strongly associated with the practice. The situation with other sexually transmitted organisms is not as clear. In seeking to find plausible reasons for such results, a number of biological phenomena have been identified—they all basically relate to the increased ease of entry of disease organisms in the uncircumcised male. There appeared to be no difference in the protection offered in Muslim and Christian countries.[365]

> *In those communities where sexual practices are maintained closer to the biblical recommendations... the incidence of cervical cancer is much lower.*

In those communities where sexual practices are maintained closer to the biblical recommendations, such as among the Amish, the incidence of cervical cancer is much lower than in surrounding communities. Similar trends may be observed among conservative Muslim women in Saudi Arabia. When a wider group of cancers are considered, conservative Christian groups (Mormons and Seventh-day Adventists) that treat the body with the utmost respect by avoiding alcohol and smoking and adopting a healthier diet also have lower cancer incidences than others. Researchers do not dismiss the possibility that family values, positive worldviews, and strong communities may also be involved. Religious practices also may positively influence the development of the fetus before it is born, such as in communities not given to the use of drugs, alcohol, cigarettes, or likely to carry sexually transmitted diseases.[366]

Highlight: Conservative religious groups that follow the scriptural recommendations connected with sexual relationships experience fewer problems from sexually transmitted diseases than other groups.

Another interesting religious tradition in Jewish and Islamic cultures is that the blood is drained from the animal (basic rule—Deuteronomy 12:16). For example, the Jews prepare kosher meat using strict guidelines. The animal is killed quickly by slitting the neck to ensure the maximum loss of blood (Leviticus 7:26, 27; 17:10–14); any injured or diseased animal is rejected (Deuteronomy 14:21—an ethical ruling even today),[367] and certain parts of the animal are considered non-kosher (sciatic nerve and adjoining blood vessels, some fat surrounding vital organs and the liver). Remaining blood is removed through the process of broiling or soaking and salting.[368] However, we must not imagine that kosher meats cannot give rise to foodborne disease. If the animals carry disease organisms and are not handled in a hygienic manner, then those who eat such foods may expect to suffer illness.[369]

In modern processing plants, kosher poultry may carry high loads of microbes on account of the multiple stages and longer processing time required, which gives the microbes time to multiply.[370] However, in strictly controlled trials, it is evident that the salting of poultry meat does significantly reduce microbe numbers over non-salted controls. Most importantly, disease organisms are reduced.[371] This should mean that on a household or small-scale level, as might have been

expected in biblical times, kosher meats were safer than traditionally prepared meat. Kosher prepared beef (meat water soaked, salted externally, and then washed), prepared in a modern setting, also showed reduced numbers of microbes including disease-causing organisms.[372] What also is certain is that kosher and halal meats are less risky products as far as degenerative nervous system disease (e.g., mad cow disease) transmission is concerned. No ill or injured animal may be slaughtered, and the method of hand slaughtering ensures that in the modern setting brain tissue does not contaminate the meat.[373]

Highlight: Meat preparation practices that involve thorough draining of blood from the carcass and a salting procedure cause a product (at least in small scale operations) to be less prone to carry high populations of disease-causing organisms.

Other practices mentioned in Scripture may also have a scientific basis. However, the examples cited are the most readily supported in today's world. The practical guidelines that I have established from selected biblical cultural and ritual practices are listed below. In other societies additional outcomes may be derived. However, in many societies measures adopted to counteract the spread of venereal diseases will of necessity go beyond the simple rules of behavior we have outlined, as those subscribing to biblical principles in the broader community represent a minority. Unfortunately, the behavior of a majority sometimes influences the health and well-being of the minority irrespective of their convictions and practice.

Guiding Principles and Practical Suggestions

1. The spread of infectious diseases may be reduced by quarantining individuals who are highly infectious and by using disinfection techniques to reduce person-to-person spread.

2. Maintenance of clean surroundings and adopting good habits of personal hygiene are necessary for the maintenance of health.

3. Disposal of human waste so as to avoid contamination of water and food sources and to prevent breeding places for flies and other vermin contributes immeasurably to the maintenance of robust human health.

4. Contamination of water and food sources with animal and human waste products leads to disease outbreaks. Proper disposal and/or treatment of these wastes are necessary to minimize the risk of human disease outbreaks. Where modern treatment facilities for these wastes are not available, the placement of disposal sites/pits is highly significant. Cross contamination with drinking water should be avoided scrupulously.

5. Items (plant or animal) that are spoiled through disease or decay processes are not suitable as food sources.

6. Meat preparation procedures that minimize contamination of carcasses with the intestinal contents and that slow microbial growth are recommended. Slowing microbial growth means keeping food at less than 4°C and at or higher than 60°C. Eating food within several hours of preparation where cooling and hot holding facilities are not available will prevent microorganisms reaching critical population levels.

7. Keeping cooked products separate from fresh materials prevents cross-contamination and problems arising from the rapid growth of microbes in cooked items.

8. Minimizing intake of blood in food products, such as in red meat, contributes positively to a reduction of the risk of contracting colorectal cancer.

9. The incidence of sexually transmitted diseases is greatly reduced when the scriptural guidelines relating to moral behavior are followed.

10. Living by the code of sexual behavior outlined in Scripture, when based on conviction, strengthens the moral fiber in the family and community and contributes to the creation of a pleasant and robust society.

11. Marriage contracts should be made carefully with some consideration being given to the genetic heritage and health of any resulting children. Contracts between close relatives and within small population groups are more likely to give rise to longevity and disability issues and may increase susceptibility to various infectious diseases.

Section II: Mental and Social Health

Memorable Quotes[374]

"Sickness is the vengeance of nature for the
violation of her laws"
(Charles Simmons).

"Joy, temperance and repose,
slam the door on the doctor's nose"
(Henry Wadsworth Longfellow).

"In a disordered mind, as in a disordered
body, soundness of health is impossible"
(Cicero).

"Harmonizing the health of body and mind
is the only way to true health"
(Hsing Yun).

"Wisdom is to the soul what
health is to the body"
(La Rochefoucauld).

"Happiness is when what you think, what you
say, and what you do are in harmony"
(Mohandas Gandhi).

"To avoid sickness eat less;
to prolong life worry less"
(Chu Hui Weng).

"O you who believe! Be patient and excel in
patience and remain steadfast,
and be careful of (your duty to) Allah,
that you may be successful"
(Koran 3:200, Shakir translation).

"Fathers, do not exasperate your children;
instead, bring them up in the training and
instruction of the Lord"
(Ephesians 6:4, NIV).

"Finally, my friends, keep your minds on
whatever is true, pure, right, holy, friendly,
and proper. Don't ever stop thinking about
what is truly worthwhile and worthy of praise"
(Philippians 4:8, CEV).

"Then Jesus said, 'Let's go off by ourselves to a
quiet place and rest awhile.'
He said this because there were so many
people coming and going that Jesus and his
apostles didn't even have time to eat"
(Mark 6:31, NLT).

Chapter 7

Intelligences of Humans

The intelligence that humans display separates them from other animals. In seeking to explain intelligence, various theories have been constructed. Tests have been devised to measure the capacity of an individual's intelligence in relation to that of others. Some believe in an overall mental capacity that regulates an individual's performance while others side with Howard Gardner and believe that individuals possess multiple, but unique, independent intelligences—e.g., logical-mathematical, musical, spatial, and so on. However, at the end of the day, the issue is how best to develop human abilities and prepare people to handle the changing circumstances of life through education.[375]

The aims of education, expressed in the United Nations documents, are to "achieve the flowering of personality" and to promote "readiness to cooperate." In order to achieve these goals, family, school, community, and nation have influential functions.[376] This UNESCO account goes on to say that group loyalties and leaders are able to influence the behavior of individuals but ultimately the behavior of a society is dependent on the stability of the bulk of society's members.[377] In times of crisis, fears are aroused and prejudices heightened, and this may lead to the rejection of sound leadership in the absence of well-informed and adjusted (emotionally competent) individuals. Thus education seeks to remove the bases for fears and prejudices and to give human beings a significant basis for cooperation and goodwill so that the dignity of all human beings will be preserved.

Family is the informal structure where education takes place. School is the formal structure designed to mold the minds of developing society members. The intellectual tasks set in the school will have a bearing on developing attitudes, but the teaching philosophy, the method, the content and the teacher's own subtle emphasis will all influence the emotional development and the values accepted by the young person. In both home and school, ideas about the equality of all, self-worth, and positive attitudes toward issues may be developed. However, in both, the absence of clear identification of issues, moral values, or the development of problem solving skills may leave the minds of children in an anxious state and hence prone to emotional abuse.

Highlight: In order to achieve the flowering of the personality, home, school, community, and nation have vital functions to perform. Clear moral values and problem solving skills are meant to be conveyed by these agencies.

Each individual brings certain possibilities for development. These abilities depend on their genetic heritage, but to a considerable extent the total environment will influence the development that actually takes place. The personalities and attitudes of the child's parents will begin the molding process and other individuals will supplement this. Security and comfort within a family or the larger group shapes behavior, as humans tend to repeat those activities that are rewarded or give satisfaction. Individuals are likely to be emotionally healthy if they learn to adjust to the changing world in which they live within a supportive environment designed to satisfy human needs. Given security, the individual is ready to accept challenges and lay aside unfounded fears and anxieties.

In such an environment, it is also possible to train the growing mind to tolerate some frustration of immediate desires so that they do not depart into unacceptable behavior (tantrums and aggression). The options offered to the child, the attitude of those who are restraining unacceptable behavior, and the way in which approval is given will determine the development of personality. The development of personality is a lifelong process. Through this process the individual will achieve acceptable behavior while satisfying both their personal aspirations and their commitment to society. The whole notion of educating for emotional health is to enable acceptable forms of behavior to be recognized and rewarded through the operation of individual initiative. Acceptable behavior is determined by each sub-culture or tradition within that society. If acceptable and unacceptable behaviors are identified in a loving, secure environment, then conformity is more likely. Such an environment will also promote human happiness.

The attitude of those who are restraining unacceptable behavior, and the way in which approval is given will determine the development of personality.

Highlight: A supportive environment in which human needs are satisfied leads to emotional health. Such an environment is characteristically loving and supportive.

In the following section, I will write briefly about the core personal skills that lead to the development of an emotionally competent approach to living.

Aspects of Competence

The aim of parents and teachers alike is to prepare those in their care to be well-adjusted individuals able to take responsibility, and possibly leadership in society, to the best of their genetic potential. Their aim is to see those in their sphere of influence prepared to work efficiently and well with others at the same time as being at peace with themselves. Robust character development is the aim according to the Christian ideal.

Parents and teachers are not alone in influencing the outcomes. All the significant groups of individuals who interact with a person can influence their developing skills. However, the influence of the childhood authority figure is of utmost importance and I will deal with this in another chapter. Other influences are brought to bear by peer groups, role models, corporate cultures (school, church, and work) and the general cultural background environment.[378]

Developing social and emotional skills is part of the rich framework that we acquire through learning. The basic elements of such learning are the ability to understand and reflect on our own emotions and appreciate and respond to the feelings of others. These competencies enable us to work through social and emotional issues.[379]

Individuals whom we call emotionally healthy are able to manage their emotions within the bounds of reason.

Individuals whom we call emotionally healthy are able to manage their emotions within the bounds of reason so that their behaviors do not overwhelm them. They are able to handle the ups and downs of life and yet still cope. A fine balance between the rational and emotional options available ensures that passions do not take control. Both types of skill influence our usefulness. Our ability to know and manage our own emotions and understand and respond to the emotions of

others is essential to our ability to get along well with others and be effective leaders. Clearly, our emotional skills can be regarded as part of our character.[380]

Highlight: *Emotionally competent individuals are able to understand their own emotions and respond appropriately to the feelings of others.*

The list of core skills that enable individuals to function with maturity may differ slightly among authors, but the following group represents one reasonably comprehensive attempt.[381] I have complemented the list with moderating comments from a Christian perspective.

Self-awareness

The term self-awareness involves both knowledge of our moods and what our thoughts are about such feelings. Those who are mindful of their moods are able to manage them more effectively. If we feel valued by others and significant and competent, this allows self-esteem (respect) to develop satisfactorily. Christian belief facilitates this state, for we are challenged to accept that we are of infinite value in God's sight (Matthew 10:29–31). The idea that we are worth something is central to personal achievement and behavior.[382]

The outpouring of outrageous love illustrated by Christ's death on the cross has established the worth of each individual.[383] What others think of an individual is viewed in this context, for believers know they are heirs of the heavenly kingdom and its riches and this will be spent in the company of Jesus Christ (Romans 8:16, 17). Such knowledge should give all great confidence.

We take feelings and previous experience into consideration when making decisions. For the Christian, gut feelings alone are an insufficient guide for action. Reference to principle is foundational to any decision. This goes beyond the virtuous attitudes generated in some confessions.[384] For the Christian, substantial and universal principles are found in moral absolutes contained in the Decalogue (Exodus 20:2–17).[385] They believe that these principles express the will of God for the human race (Psalm 40:8). At their center these guidelines are meant to protect the relationships that really matter in life—namely, our relationship to God (first four principles) and our relationship to one another (last six principles).[386]

Highlight: All individuals are of equal and infinite value on account of Christ's sacrifice. Such a realization gives a sense of purpose and destiny.

Self-control

Controlling one's emotions and adapting to changing circumstances is foundational to emotional skill. Solomon, reportedly the wisest man to live in the ancient Eastern world, tells us that we should not be in a hurry to express anger, as this is the way taken by foolish people. His father advised all diligently to control their wrath, for "*it* only causes harm" (Psalm 37:8; cf. Ecclesiastes 7:9). This agrees with the Chinese proverb that says: "Patience in a moment of anger can save you a thousand days of pain." Indeed, this sentiment also was expressed by the great Christian apostle Paul some two thousand years ago. His advice was get anger under control quickly; certainly "do not let the sun go down" before you settle the matter (Ephesians 4:26). Emotional peace is the key to a pleasant life. Current medical advice agrees with the counsel of our ancient sources, and we do well not to relive our unpleasant experiences again and again.[387]

When emotions are out of control for too long, health and well-being are adversely affected. Those given to acute episodes of anger are many times more likely to trigger a heart attack as those who have their emotions under control.[388] We may attempt to manage emotions by what we do, read, listen to, or view. Most would agree whole-heartedly that we should be temperate in all things,

including our emotions. This is advice that all great athletes practice in order to realize success; a similar undertaking is needed by all who would live a successful life (1 Corinthians 9:25). In fact, those who believe in a Supreme Helper, such as Christians, hold that everything that a person does should be done with a view to bringing "glory to God" (1 Corinthians 10:31). This is indeed a superior motivating idea.

Factors motivating individuals to show determined self-control are varied. Cultural expectations may demand such behavior or the desire for the rewards available to upwardly mobile people may be a great motivator. A much higher motivation force activates the Christian's thinking. Such recognize that human life was created by God and that each individual's existence has direction and purpose. In the present world, the purpose is to be stewards of God's creation, to share the knowledge of His saving love with others, and to work productively in the society in which they find themselves. A Christian is motivated by the reality of God's presence and His promises, the unbreakable pulling power of God's love expressed in the life, death, and continuing ministry of Christ, and the promise of being with Him in the earth made new (Romans 4:21, 8:37–39; 1 Thessalonians 4:13–18; Revelation 21:1–4). When individuals understand that their lives have a high purpose, they are more willing to labor under varying circumstances until the great plan of God has been fulfilled in their lives. In every circumstance, they can set worthy goals and be confident of God's blessing.

Highlights:

1. Control of the emotions leads both to good health and happy relationships.

2. The motivation to self-control is strong for Christians for they understand the high purpose of God for their lives.

Self-motivation

Enthusiasm, persistence, and confidence are associated consistently with success, so also is the idea of deferred gratification in pursuit of a goal. The ability to resist impulse or temptation now in order to gain a future reward is strongly associated with social competence and personal effectiveness. An optimistic, hopeful view of life also allows difficult challenges to be accepted and conquered consistently. Both these qualities can be improved through learning.

Those who believe in the Christian philosophy do not have particular difficulties with motivation because the foundations of their belief are saturated in optimism and hope (Romans 8:17; 1 John 3:2, 3). This motivates them to live a life of devoted service to God and His principles here. The love that God has shown for human beings in dying overwhelms hearers so much that obedience is a joyful experience. Hope experienced in the spiritual dimension of an individual's life will spill over into everyday living. For example, a hopeful attitude in life leads to persistence in achieving goals. Those who are hopeful have an advantage in life; they are simply more successful.[389]

An optimistic view of life is a motivating force for individuals.

An optimistic view of life is a motivating force for individuals. Christians should be able to look beyond the difficulties and disappointments of life to the future (John 16:33). For them life is not a game of chance, as indicated by the theory of evolution.[390] Personal failures do not make Christians helpless. They respond positively, knowing that there is appropriate advice in God's Word and that divine help is at hand. The challenge is to catch some of the optimism displayed by the apostle Paul.

He said, "For I am convinced that neither death nor life, neither angels nor demons, neither the present nor the future, nor any powers, neither height nor depth, nor anything else in all creation, will be able to separate us from the love of God that is in Christ Jesus our Lord" (Romans 8:38, 39, NIV).

Now, the impact of the mental attitude and approach to life on physical health is profound. The body mounts attacks on disease organisms through the immune system, which is more vigorous in optimistic people. Then, too, these individuals have a positive attitude toward changing lifestyle practices; they are more likely to approach life's issues creatively, and they have more friends to support them in their time of need. All this aids toward a favorable outcome.[391]

Highlights:

1. Enthusiasm, confidence, and persistence are associated with success as is deferred gratification.

2. A hopeful and optimistic approach to life helps in achieving goals. Christians are able to show both qualities in abundance.

3. The body's immune system response is heightened by positive attitudes, and this contributes to good health.

Empathy

The ability to sense the feelings of others is the basis for a caring, mature attitude—such individuals possess emotional competence. Entering into the distress of others leads one to come to their help. Empathy is set in a moral framework. For instance, when a person is wronged, the tendency with many is to spring to their defense.[392] A substantive basis for showing empathy is a realization that all human beings are equal before God and were created in the image of their creator, making human beings different to all other living beings

(Genesis 1:27; John 3:16). The idea that there is a God who loves every person and is not a torturer of those who fall short of His requirements effectively extinguishes fear.[393] There is no fear in love (Psalm 34:7; 1 John 4:18).

Social Skills

The ability to establish relationships is at the root of the individual's effectiveness with others. Socially adept people can express emotions, are empathetic, and can lead and organize. Essentially they are emotionally mature and build on these skills to work with others. They sense, understand, and react appropriately to other people's emotions and understand the dynamics of the group.[394] I will explore this area more extensively in the study on social conscience.

In the following sections, I deal with some of the additional strategies adopted by mature individuals that assist in coping with changing circumstances.

Focusing on Change

Few individuals living in our modern world can complete their lives without experiencing change and confronting arresting events. These episodes may be as common as changing jobs, falling ill, or getting married, but may be more complex, such as having to live in a community racked with hatred and violence. As individuals, we respond to these and other changes in various ways.

The manner in which we respond to events occurring around us is dependent on many factors. For a limited few, their genetic heritage will be first in importance in determining their response. The majority, however, respond in ways determined by the total life experience. This experience is conditioned by family, school, and community interactions and the value system that they have acquired.

Some of the most fascinating and challenging accounts of how individuals handle change come

from those who have experienced disabling accidents or are born disabled. If we focus momentarily on the life of Louise Sauvage, a highly decorated Australian Paralympian, we notice the importance of personal attitudes, family, friends, and the broader community in shaping her life. Although born with a congenital disability, she commenced competing at age eight and did so with determination. When offered a chance to feature in the Barcelona Olympics, the help and cooperation of her family and friends were vital to her success.[395] We would resoundingly classify Louise's attitude and approach to life as mature and inspiring.

It is the idea of maturity in our approach to life's events that we will explore briefly. When looking at this subject, it is well to recognize that peoples' response to events depends on personality traits. Behavior is also driven by needs or by goals. Many individuals choose to take less enjoyable detour pathways in pursuit of the long-term objectives.[396] Maturity is not only indicated by goal setting but also involves the ability to understand ourselves and others and to work cooperatively with our work companions. Our ability to understand ourselves and others defines our mental well-being.[397]

Highlight: Individuals who hold reasonably well-defined short- and long-term goals are regarded characteristically as mature and they inspire others.

Characteristics of a Mature Approach to Living

All appreciate well-adjusted individuals, but when asked to identify those features that have led to this conclusion we may differ in our opinions. One abbreviated list is suggested below.[398]

Constructive Approach

Those who cope best with events taking place around them accept the reality of the issues confronting them and explore avenues of possible resolution. The solutions may reside in the person's own resources or may be found elsewhere. Sometimes we might be blinded to significant issues and need help from others with a different perspective.[399] No reasonable option is ignored. The well-balanced individual also does not ignore or try to escape the issue and does not worry excessively. Those engaged in a constructive approach will accept their role in the process of betterment and will put effort into achieving an improved outcome.

An example of such an approach might be cited from the biblical record. Queen Esther (a Jewess) found herself in a most awkward situation when a high court official proposed to King Ahasuerus (Xerxes) that the Jewish race should be eliminated or severely reduced (Esther 3:8–13). She attempted to implement a constructive approach to resolve the issue, under her cousin's suggestion (Esther 4:4–17). This was so effective that the grand designer of the scheme was neutralized and ethnic cleansing did not occur (Esther 7).

Ability to Adapt

In our rapidly moving world, we all appreciate the necessity for altering our approach and plans to take changing circumstances in stride. This is not a matter of making change for change sake, but represents the ability to adapt, to innovate, and to remain gracious about our changing circumstances.

Paul of Tarsus was never one to feel helpless about changing circumstances.

Well-adjusted individuals have understood this throughout time. A good illustration from the historical records relates to the man also known as Paul of Tarsus living around two thousand years ago. He was never one to feel helpless about changing circumstances. This attitude allowed him to

adapt the communication of his philosophical beliefs in a sensitive manner. The record informs us that he met a group of philosophers (Stoics and Epicureans) on Mars' Hill in Athens, Greece. His principal aim was to share the good news that Christ died for all in an overwhelming expression of love and that all are dependent on God for very existence. In order to convey these concepts, he used the wording on an altar inscription to the UNKNOWN GOD and the well-known lines from the peoples' poet to excite interest—"For we are His offspring," he said (Acts 17:22–34). In other words, he adapted his approach to the worldview of the people so they would consider his ideas favorably. This is an effective approach to ministry with people holding different outlooks.

We can be certain that in adapting to various situations that he always gave attention to principle as a rule of life. This is shown in his rebuke of the apostle Peter at a later time. Peter was embarrassed by ethnic prejudices and failed to follow principle. Paul urged him, and by example us, to put principle as the guiding star in all our decision-making (Galatians 2:11–21).

Short and Long-Term Goals

The idea of goals was raised in our first point, but requires a little expansion. I might illustrate by referring again to our sporting hero, Louise Sauvage. She had short-term goals, which were conceivably attainable through hard work, and at the same time she had long-term aspirations not connected with personal sporting achievement.[400] Louise focused first on short-term goal setting, but at the same time she was willing to make sacrifices in order to give greater chances for her aspirations to succeed in the long run. The idea of sacrificing in the short term to make long-term gains is a characteristic of the mature individual.

This idea has been around for a long time. There is a story related in Eastern folklore about day workers waiting at the employment agency for work. Each potential worker was trying to meet short-term goals by earning money from day work. Some seeking work were fortunate to be employed all day, others were less fortunate and were employed for a short period of time. Those who commenced to work in the field an hour before finishing time reasonably expected to be paid accordingly. They were surprised when they received a day's wages. Their short-term goals were exceeded. Willingness to risk something was the important starting point. Their attitude toward the other workers, who had been employed all day, is another element in explaining the rewards they received (Matthew 20:1–16). They were undoubtedly optimists and were determined to avoid adopting a helpless attitude.

There is an Eastern parable told in some communities about our natural abilities and how we should use them. The story has it that an employer went on a journey to a distant country and delegated different levels of responsibility to his employees, giving them strict instructions to show initiative and increase his profit margins. When he returned most had taken advantage of their responsibilities, but one individual had done nothing but rather preferred to blame the employer's attitude and methods of operation as excuses for being unproductive. This individual was severely punished, but the others were honored (Matthew 25:14–30). The story tells us that our attitude influences the extent of our effort and has a bearing on the outcome. An optimist focuses on potential success, not on the negatives that may be present. The wise counsel of the Bible is that "whatever your hand finds to do, do it with your might" (Ecclesiastes 9:10). We carefully note that the parable does not condemn those who cannot find employment opportunities.

Long-term goals are significant to Christians, as the apostle Paul summarized in the words: "For I am persuaded that neither death nor life … nor things present nor things to come … shall be able to separate us from the love of God…." (Romans 8:38, 39). This optimistic view of the future is based on the love of God and His trustworthiness. The perception of God's ability to deliver is based on both personal experience and the formidable record of fulfilled prophecies.[401]

Optimism is an attitude that has intrigued the medical profession in recent years because it promotes a faster and better recovery after surgery. One of the reasons for this is that optimists refuse to be helpless; they try and make a difference. This mental attitude has an effect on the whole body, such that it is better able to fight disease and repair itself after an operation.[402] I will say more on this topic in later chapters.

Team Player but Capable of Independence

Sharing time and ideas with others is essential for the development of mutual good will and trust. The ability to think well or considerately of other peoples' opinions does not clash with the idea of independent thought and action. Each type of action has its place. The ability to make decisions and move ahead in confidence is the hallmark of those who have reached maturity. In our first section (Aspects of Competence), I touched briefly on the significance of social skills. Here I expand on these a little.

Exchanging ideas from different perspectives is the high point of teamwork, and there are other benefits.[403] The early Christian church located at Jerusalem grasped the significance of group discussion and cooperation as it grappled with the growth of the church among diverse ethnic groups—it grew as a result (Acts 15:6–29). Experiences and concerns were shared and discussed by the church leaders and an agreed broad approach was taken to maintain unity. Within this framework, individual enthusiasm and initiative could be expressed in the full knowledge that general approval of a joint position would come from the group. Indeed, there is a beautiful picture sketched by the apostle Paul. He conceives of the ideal church as a well-coordinated body—all its members function in a complementary manner to give strength and direction to the group endeavor (1 Corinthians 12:12–31). This principle applies to society, work-related issues, and the family. Independent and cooperative behaviors toward a common goal make for satisfying outcomes.

Team values can be taught.[404] In fact, one of the plagues devastating modern society is the pursuit of individual interests. Modernization as experienced in the Western world has brought this emphasis to the fore and breeds a "culture of separation." The manner in which individual choice is exercised and managed in various democratic nations varies widely and may be far from satisfactory. One strategy that would halt this downward slide is a worldview that involves coherent moral and intellectual ideas. The good news is that this is exactly what can be experienced in some religious communities operating within the broader community.[405]

Well-adjusted individuals control their emotions and show impartiality toward others. They are emotionally competent. These ideas have been dealt with broadly in a previous section, but I wish to express some additional thoughts under several headings.

Control of Emotions

Emotions are part of healthy existence. Loss of emotional control by some of our sports and film stars fixes them forever in our minds as challenged and disqualifies them from being positive role models. In addition, the mature person shows a refusal to dwell excessively on the negative aspects of life and is able to move past disappointments, frustration, and fears and focuses on the positive.

It has long been held in certain communities that there is a time to express the emotions common to humanity (Ecclesiastes 3:1, 4). If we take grief as our example, the expression of this emotion allows the individual to work through the issues and move on. Take the death of a friend or companion as the event. Through the expression of grief, the individual is able to show respect for the loved one and to re-establish their own independence within a framework of empathy and active help. A significant issue is that through this experience the individual must be encouraged by those supporting them in order to maintain self-esteem (respect), self-worth, and confidence; hence, minimizing the possibility for descent into depression.[406]

The mature person shows a refusal to dwell excessively on the negative aspects of life

Anger and hostility are emotions that are worth saying something about. Both are good predictors of increased risk of death from coronary heart disease.[407] A fascinating recent study has shown that individuals devoted to a plant-based diet experience fewer negative emotions than meat eaters.[408] The advice from an ancient king (David) is "Stop being angry! Turn from your rage! Do not lose your temper—it only leads to harm" (Psalm 37:8, NLT). He no doubt was aware of the God-given diet in Eden. Adopting it is good counsel and will promote long life.

Concern and Love for Others

The ability to love others, irrespective of race, color, or religion is something that most value highly (e.g., Mahatma Gandhi, Martin Luther King, and Mother Teresa). In everyday terms such concern translates as gracious acceptance of the views and aspirations of others as being important. These views will not be sacrificed wantonly to further one's own egotistical visions.

I have already introduced the subject of empathy, but we need to make some additional comments. Empathetic feelings and prosocial acts (sharing, caring, comforting acts) are valued almost universally, but they need to be fostered in children, for environmental influences can suppress them. Persons living in industrialized societies are under particular disadvantages, for the idea of everyone contributing to the family welfare is not as strongly developed as in many less privileged societies. This is perhaps on account of competition being more highly valued in industrialized societies than in some other groups. Nevertheless, parents who are warm and think of others themselves can aid their children taking on the same values by verbal reinforcement of cooperative, sharing behavior. Children are more likely to practice things they hear if the person making the speech practices what they say.[409]

Concern for others is one thing, but we may question how it is possible to love those who may be disagreeable (Matthew 22:38–40; 1 John 4:20). The well-known apostle Paul fortunately explains the process for Christians. He said that "the love of Christ compels us" (2 Corinthians 5:14). In other words, it is possible only as each person responds to the love that God has shown toward them. It is submitted that the only reasonable response to God's outrageous expression of unselfish love is absolute devotion to Him and, as a result, the individual acts as a channel for His love to flow to others. God's love (*agape*) is not a natural part of the human experience. As we come to understand and know God, it is possible for us to be channels for His love. When we act in this fashion, the focus for our kindness is our neighbor, not on any benefit that we may gain through the helpful act done.[410]

Productivity

The final, and generally agreed, measure of maturity is the ability to effectively perform tasks and be productive. Those who are not coping spend considerable time and effort planning or actually trying to undertake a task and yet making little progress in task fulfillment or doing it poorly.

Christians, if they accept their philosophy fully, will take notice of one of the great figures in their history. The apostle Peter urged believers to be alert in mind or be "mentally stripped for action" (1 Peter 1:13–16, NEB). This is on account of the fact that the task of living in an unwholesome world according to the principles of God's Word is a serious business. We cannot afford to fill the mind with the impure, the violent, and the silly (1 Chronicles 28:9; Psalm 101:3; Philippians 4:8). Modern means of communication specialize in occupying time with endless images that can pervert the mind and keep it from productive activities.

Highlight: *Mature individuals are emotionally competent and have the ability to set goals, work creatively and productively with others, adapt, and show great emotional control and concern for others.*

Guiding Principles and Practical Suggestions

1. Education seeks to remove the bases for fears and prejudices and to give human beings a significant basis for cooperation and goodwill so that the dignity of all will be preserved.

2. Individuals are likely to be emotionally healthy if they learn to adjust to the changing world in which they live within a supportive environment designed to satisfy human needs.

3. Acceptable and unacceptable behavior identified in a loving, secure environment is more likely to be assimilated by young people.

4. Emotionally healthy individuals are able to manage their emotions within the bounds of reason so that their behaviors do not overwhelm them. They have self-awareness,

self-control, self-motivation, empathy, and social skills.

5. Attitudes promoting emotional maturity are that fears are restricted and prejudices are eliminated through education, discussion, and guided experiences.

6. Those who cope best with events taking place around them accept the reality of the issues confronting them and explore avenues of possible resolution. They adopt a constructive approach. Well-adjusted individuals have the ability to adapt, innovate, and remain gracious about changing circumstances.

7. Short-term goal setting is significant in the lives of well-adjusted individuals, but at the same time they are willing to make sacrifices in order to give greater chances for long-term satisfaction.

8. Sharing time and ideas with others is essential for the development of mutual good will and trust. The ability to think well or considerately of other peoples' opinions does not clash with the idea of independent thought and action.

9. The mature person shows a refusal to dwell excessively on the negative aspects of life and is able to move past disappointments, frustration, and fears and focuses on the positive.

10. The ability to love others, irrespective of race, color, or religion is a principle expressed by those actively concerned about the well-being and happiness of others. This may translate as gracious acceptance of their views and aspirations.

11. A well-recognized measure of maturity is the ability to effectively perform tasks and be productive. These people are active in both thinking and doing.

Chapter 8

Planets in Cooperation

John Gray's assertion that men and women are as different as inhabitants from Mars and Venus is currently under heavy challenge with strong evidence developing that there are more similarities than differences between the sexes. This means that personality, cognitive ability, and leadership are basically similar with some differences noted in motor skills, sexuality, and aggression. The emphasis now has turned to the influence of social roles on behavior.[411]

Families classically are made of a man and a woman with a variable number of children. These are units that provide love, interest, discipline, and security to the growing child. They have been vilified in the immediate past for a number of reasons. Some see families as oppressive and contributing to mental illness, others as a place where women are marginalized and denied freedom. We can add to this list those who find the private domain (of which families are a part) competing with the interests of powerful institutions in the public domain. Finally, in our market driven world, some merely treat families as commodities.[412]

Added to this pressure, the nature of families is being redefined as society accepts different arrangements. In Western societies the traditional nuclear family was one where the father was the major provider and the mother the major caregiver. Such families are now in the minority with a more egalitarian structure being favored. Dual income families are on the increase in these societies as are single parent families. The latter trend is due mainly to divorce. The end result of these and other changes is that the significance of the family as a demographic reality has declined. Non-family groups are on the increase. In addition, the cohesion of families, the strength of its social functions, and the influence of families in society have decreased.[413]

While some of the criticisms of exploitation in the family can be supported by scientific evidence and personal experience, there are certain types of families that give their participants stability and resilience and contribute much to the achievement of intellectual and social efficiency in children. It is to these families that I will direct our attention. Family life can be the most rewarding experience and is the place where moral values, worldview, social concerns, and creative approaches to life issues are developed.[414]

Successful parenting ideally commences at birth.

Successful parenting ideally commences at birth. Mothers given access to their babies immediately after birth and on a daily basis while in the hospital develop a strong bond with their children. The bond is evident in the early years in that immediate contact mothers show more affectionate behavior and a richer verbal interaction with their babies than do mothers whose initial contact is delayed and restricted. It is believed by some that infants show the benefits of such bonding in performance on language and intelligence tests. Early childhood development in social, intellectual, and linguistic skills is also related to parenting style. Such a style is not dependent on cultural or economic factors. Interested individuals can learn a good parenting style; the benefits are measurable and continue well beyond preschool.[415] Infants who show robust attachment to their caregiver (through affectionate and sensitive caregiving) at the age of one year are more resilient and show superior problem solving and

social skills in preschool than those children who do not have sound attachments. In secure, warm families, infants are also attached to fathers, who tend to be outgoing, agreeable, and happy.[416]

Attempts by the public education system to minimize the impact of social and family background on student competencies largely have been unsuccessful so that the inequalities existing in the student population at the commencement of schooling are evident when they exit school life. Studies have indicated that family background and attitudes have a major impact on achievement right through the school years. Parents in the habit of reading to their children and enriching their educational experiences exerted a positive influence on educational attainment outcomes. Parental interest in the progress of the child is also significant. Factors such as curriculum, facilities, and especially teacher's characteristics and expectations do impact achievement. However, there is no substitute for parental interest and encouragement so that children gain the greatest benefit from their school experience. The likelihood of children moving counter to family achievement expectations or breaking with established norms and routines to enable achievement to happen is not particularly high. With the growth of one-parent families, the question of progress at school is of some interest. If the remaining parent shows interest and there is an absence of conflict, progress can be maintained. The preferable state is a stable family structure with supportive processes in place to give children the greatest chance of developing their competencies.[417]

Highlight: *A strong mother-child bond established immediately after birth and positive family attitudes and encouragement aid in student achievement.*

Families and Health

The health of the individual is inextricably linked to family experiences either past or present.

These experiences impact emotional, mental, and physical health. The processes most frequently observed in families that promote the establishment of competent members are as follows.[418]

Communication Patterns

The quality and characteristics of communication are vital to successful family life. This has been appreciated by many for a long time. Such understanding is clearly outlined in a delightful piece of writing coming from the pen of an ancient sage telling of his joy at hearing his loved one speak (Song of Solomon 2:10–14). Solomon, a wise man from the East, said in speaking of his spouse: "Let me hear your voice, for your voice *is* sweet, and your face *is* lovely" (verse 14). The remainder of the book from which this quotation comes gives no doubt that the relationship between the two individuals being spoken of was most fulfilling. A successful family relationship also shows a constant and comfortable place for empathy. The ability to respond to the feelings of others is critical to the alleviation of marital stress; its absence is a major contributor to marital breakdown.[419] In fact, Jesus, around whose birth modern time is calculated in many countries, showed the importance of empathy to His followers and admirers through example. This feature of His character was shown by His simple response following contact with a close family group who had lost a member in death. The record simply says: "Jesus wept" (John 11:35).

Failure to communicate effectively can lead to very distressing outcomes and is highlighted in another story which comes to us from Eastern lore that may be known by many. The people featured in the famous story were Rebecca and Isaac. Now, there were favorites among their children, and this was especially evident with their twin sons: Esau and Jacob. The first son was due to receive the birthright by the custom of the time, but he did not appreciate his spiritual responsibilities and privileges. Jacob, on the other hand, earnestly desired the privileges that his brother scorned. The parents failed to communicate effectively about the issues, leading to deception being practiced on the father and a sad history of family dispute followed in which Jacob was forced to flee in danger of his life (Genesis 27:1–45).

Clear communications directed at the person in question rather than vague instructions given casually or by inference are desirable in the area of task allocation. Communication of feelings and emotions are equally important and should be given with the same clarity, with frequent indications of individual wants, needs, and opinions. Effective communication also involves active listening to children and responding in ways that validate and guide rather than accuse and discourage. In healthier families, a wide range of feelings can be expressed without the possibility of personal criticism or angry outbursts occurring. Comments are moderated and explanatory, not unkind and destructive. There is genuine empathy among the members. In such families, positions are explained in warmth, love, and consistency and, as a consequence, compliance with requests is more likely to occur. Families that communicate effectively tend to be resilient; they cope with crises more effectively.[420] This is the type of behavior that the prophet Isaiah pictured as being modeled by the Supreme God of the universe in relation to His subjects here on earth (Isaiah 1:18).

Families that communicate effectively tend to be resilient; they cope with crises more effectively.

The practice of confirming another person's opinion is important as it indicates that the individual is noticed and valued. Positive appreciation of others in the family group is also a significant factor in reinforcing self-image and self-confidence. Such praise is for genuine contributions and achievement. It is thought that expressions of affirmation, love, and support exert a singular influence on children's self-esteem.[421] The question of positive affirmation and appreciation in maintaining family relations is brought to our attention by the apostle Paul who made startling predictions of conditions in families near the close of earth's history. He predicted that a time would arrive when people would love themselves and focus on wealth, be full of praise of their own accomplishments, and be dismissive of things relating to others and the heavenly realm. In such an environment of selfishness, he asserted that children would grow up and become disobedient to parents and family relationships would suffer. A climate featuring a lack of thankfulness, love, and forgiveness would develop. Instead of self-control, goodness, and gentleness, headstrong and even brutal behavior would be shown together with a decided lack of appreciation for the holy or spiritual aspects of existence (2 Timothy 3:1–5). The individuals pictured in this prophecy did not express appreciation in their families or show respect for the opinions of others. Some today might argue that these very features are well developed in the society in which they live!

Both affirmation and appreciation are essential for the establishment of confidence and a positive self-image. Both these also are vital ingredients to the development of healthy family and society members.[422] However, flattery and blind affection do not contribute to a robust family or societal structure (Psalm 12:1–4). It is a form of dishonest manipulation.[423]

In healthy families, issues requiring discussion or positions that are disputed are raised at an appropriate time and resolved quickly so as to restore harmony. The process by which issues are resolved is significant. Today's modern communication experts would agree with the advice given many years ago by King Solomon who said: "A soft answer turns away wrath, but a harsh word stirs up anger. The tongue of the wise uses knowledge rightly, but the mouth of the fool pours forth foolishness" (Proverbs 15:1, 2). This is something that, if practiced, would reduce the world's family miseries. The general principles by which Christians are advised to operate their interpersonal relationships are spoken of clearly by the famous apostle Paul and are worth quoting. He puts the standard at a high level as follows: "Let all bitterness, wrath, anger, clamor, and evil speaking be put away from you, with all malice. And be kind to one another, tenderhearted, forgiving one another, even as God in Christ forgave you" (Ephesians 4:31, 32; cf. Romans 12:10; Ephesians 6:4). In other words, kindness is the "in" word; all other forms of response are clearly in forbidden territory. Now it should not be strange to learn that the ability to express feelings without criticizing or verbally attacking others is the pattern of behavior mastered by healthy families. The pattern of behavior adopted by competent parents is one of supporting growth, developing competencies, and providing children with opportunities to contribute and accept responsibility. They discipline their children in order to develop beautiful characters.[424]

In the context of disagreements, perhaps I need to mention a few words about optimism. The future well-being of children is linked to an optimistic approach to life and living. Our initial impressions or those of our children's may be incorrect. The process of broadening options and challenging initial fears is at the heart of an optimistic lifestyle. A parent may gently challenge a child's reactions and show them that there are other ways of seeing the events around them. If this approach is reinforced by the parent's response to challenging circumstances, the optimistic approach is reinforced.[425] One of the most respected prophets who lived in ancient times (Samuel) encouraged all to be optimistic. He advised that the response to changing circumstances might be a statement of confidence. His choice of words was: "'Thus far the Lord has helped us'" (1 Samuel 7:12).

Jesus gave a good example to parents in His response to His mother's rebuke. Readers will remember that as a twelve-year-old boy He had stayed behind to discuss theology with the teachers in the temple in Jerusalem after His parents had left the Passover. His mother rebuked Him about failing to inform them of His activities in the words "why have You done this to us?" His gentle response was that she should have been more aware of His growing realization of God's purpose for His life (Luke 2:46–49). The take-home message to readers is that parents should be sensitive to the changing needs and aspirations of their children. This would bring both flexibility and optimism into their management strategy.

Highlights:

1. *Clear communication patterns and the expression of empathy are foundational to healthy and resilient families.*

2. *Affirmation and appreciation of family members and the display of mutual respect lead to the development of confidence and positive feelings of self.*

3. *In healthy families, disputed issues are resolved quickly with kindness and a note of optimism introduced.*

Use of Power

In well-adjusted families, decision-making power is shared. This may be within the traditional gender role structure or outside it. However, this does not matter as long as the assumed roles are considered fair and reasonable by the family. The ideal relationship involves mutual dependence and cooperation between spouses. This is the way of love (1 Corinthians 13:4, 5). Now love will

not develop where domination and submission are the norm. In healthy families, an effective, loving "parental coalition" is evident with power not being exercised in a domineering way either between the spouses or with the children.[426]

> *In healthy families, an effective, loving "parental coalition" is evident with power not being exercised in a domineering way.*

A remarkable word picture of a virtuous woman has been left for our consideration by King Lemuel's mother (Proverbs 31). It is worth recording in part, as follows: "Who can find a virtuous wife? For her worth *is* far above rubies. The heart of her husband safely trusts her; so he will have no lack of gain. She does him good and not evil all the days of her life. She seeks wool and flax, and willingly works with her hands. She is like the merchant ships, she brings her food from afar. She also rises while it is yet night, and provides food for her household, and a portion for her maidservants. She considers a field and buys it; from her profits she plants a vineyard" (verses 10–16). This account shows that the wife had a vital part in the power sharing arrangement in the household highlighted. In fact, the entire family operation would have become dysfunctional without her input, and the husband was acutely aware of this (verses 27, 28). Of course, the view presented here and elsewhere in Scripture is that, in the cultures spoken about, leadership among equals was given to the male (Ephesians 5:22; cf. Genesis 3:16).

The use of threats or punishments is minimal in healthy families. Effective parents take a clear stand on issues from the early years; they accept their authority roles. There is minimal use of authoritarian power, and they encourage the young to make decisions within bounds that are clearly understood and reasonable. The parents are in control, setting routines and norms of behavior, with fathers playing a decisive role. The increase of freedom in decision-making on the approach of adolescence is safe, for these children have internalized parental values in a supportive environment.[427] This modern view of the use of power has its ancient counterparts. Christian parents are peacekeepers (Matthew 5:9). The norm is to give encouragement through instruction and reason while resorting to punishment only where words have proved ineffective. Such an approach will give positive and satisfying results (Proverbs 22:6, 15).

Highlights:

1. *In healthy families decision-making power is shared in a loving parental coalition.*

2. *The bounds of acceptable behavior are clearly understood through reasoned explanation. Family guidelines are maintained with minimal recourse to threats and punishment.*

Support Networks

The support network that may be available for accessing first is the extended family. In Eastern cultures and less developed nations, extended family structures are generally much more important than in the West. Such combinations may include the in-laws as well as grandparents.[428] Beyond the family, access to networks of support (peer groups, friends, or community groups), whether in the emotional or material domains, help family members to gain better opinions of themselves and to cope with the difficulties of parenting or just life itself. Some ancient and modern societies have discovered that such networks are particularly helpful. In Christian society (church), soon after the beginning of the present era, a community help-group came into existence in the city of Joppa (modern day Jaffa in Israel). The woman

who organized this was Dorcas who made coats and garments for needy widows (Acts 9:36–39). On account of the benefits that such groups give, this practice has been continued in certain communities into modern times.[429]

In Christian communities, members are encouraged to address questions of dispute among themselves in a kind and systematic manner rather than calling for the services of the legal profession and holding their faith to ridicule (1 Corinthians 6:5–8). Taking group responsibility in such a manner is not done in an attempt to hide from the civil law (Romans 13:1–3), but in order to gain sound advice from those who have had successful human relationships. Many other types of groups are available in some societies to help individuals recovering from certain diseases and for those who have children with special needs.[430]

The support of community members in transmitting moral values is also highly significant. Those societies that deliberately foster moral values through the schooling system, because they represent group values, are successful in transmitting socially mature ideals to the young. In contrast, those societies that argue values are not appropriately taught in public school have reaped the fruit in producing antisocial children.[431]

Highlights:

1. *Support networks based on family, community help groups, and faith-communities aid families to cope with many issues.*

2. *Faith-based schooling systems allow families to find support and assistance in transmission to children of understandings regarding social responsibility and moral values.*

Family Time

Time provided together to communicate, make decisions, and enjoy each other's company is vital to healthy family functioning. This means gaining control over TV exposure, computer games, club activities, and the like so that the time with the family is not compromised. Eating meals in front of the television screen is particularly damaging to communication and the development of close family relationships. Other negative effects of this practice are that the intake of fruits and vegetable declines and there may be a tendency to show weight gains.[432]

In the pressured societies in which we live, the temptation is overwhelming for some to devote more and more time to business, academic, or career success. This results in the reduction of quality time with the family and also contributes to marriage failure. We need more fathers like Daniel Petre. He stepped back from his successful career and considered the impact of his lifestyle on the family. Daniel showed early promise at Microsoft Corporation and rapidly rose through the ranks to vice president at the Seattle headquarters. But instead of continuing to relish the label of someone going somewhere in a hurry, he chose to work more intelligently and to reject the obsessive work ethic in the corporate world to return to a lower level job so that he could devote more time and attention to his family, thereby becoming a more "full and complete human being."[433] By devoting time to our children, we make them feel appreciated and special, and we contribute to the development of strength of character and give them assurance that they have worth and dignity and are loved.[434]

This response is similar to the one that the prophet Malachi, living four centuries before the present era, called for. He foresaw a time coming when family breakdown would be commonplace. He considered that the commitment of fathers to their families would be particularly rewarding in reversing this trend (Malachi 4:5, 6). In addition to this good advice, humanity's Creator commenced a practice just after He made the first human pair to assist in the development and maintenance of strong family bonds. He instructed the human family to make a commitment of time in which spiritual instruction and family togetherness would take place on a regular basis. He specified the seventh day as the divinely chosen rest day (Sabbath), as this had the value of acknowledging both His creative and salvation gifts (Exodus 20:8–11; cf. Mark 2:27). This means that the Sabbath (Saturday) is a special time in which to develop family and divine relationships. We should treasure the opportunity that God has provided.

Highlights:

1. *Time spent with the family is both self-fulfilling and creates family cohesion.*

2. *Humanity's Creator set aside a day (Saturday) for family togetherness and spiritual renewal.*

Spousal Bond

The strength of the family depends on the ability of spouses to communicate, trust, love, and function in harmony. According to Dr. Eastman, a strong personal bond has "the power to protect the family" from adverse external events.[435] There is a delightful word picture in Jewish literature that outlines close to an ideal relationship. It is described by the sage Solomon as follows: "You have ravished my heart, my sister, *my* spouse; you have ravished my heart. With one *look* of your eyes, with one link of your necklace. How fair is your love, my sister, *my* spouse! How much better than wine is your love, and the scent of your perfumes than all spices! Your lips, O *my* spouse, drip as the honeycomb; honey and milk *are* under your tongue; and the fragrance of your garments *is* like the fragrance of Lebanon" (Song of Solomon 4:9–11).

The strength of the bond shown by the couple pictured in our quote is unquestioned and represents God's ideal, for the whole book written by Solomon is also an allegory of the relationship between God and His church. There is no substitute for a strong, positive relationship between spouses to ensure emotional and intellectual development in children. Where a strong coalition exists, leadership roles are shared, authoritarian behavior is not exercised, and the partners complement each other's skills. The closeness of the bond determines the "quality of total family life."[436]

Highlight: *A strong spouse bond assists emotional and intellectual development in children.*

Religious and Spiritual Traditions and Rituals

Religious and spiritual rituals are associated with healthy families. A belief system enables members to cope with loss within the supporting framework of a community of caring individuals. One strong example of such a ritual is behavior associated with death, which differs among societies. This event in the Christian context is not meant to be a time to express abject grief and a future without hope. It is meant to be a time of memories and warm encouragement of those who have lost their loved one. The Christian church network gives a sense of belonging and purpose and allows family members to deal with loss and grief more effectively than those who do not have a belief system or a basis for hope beyond death (1 Thessalonians 4:13–18). The basis of the Christian hope is eternal life with God in His new world free from suffering and sin and where justice and love are the norm. Such beliefs give positive outcomes (including physical health) in coping with stressful situations.[437]

In many countries in Asia, cultural traditions dictate that loyal and feeling family members will express filial piety to the departed parent by performing various ceremonies on a regular basis. The Bible is very clear that respect, obedience, and reverence to parents is our Christian duty (Exodus 20:12; Ephesians 6:1–3). The mutual respect between parents and children is based on God's love. In reality honoring parents might be thought of as an expression of worship and of giving honor to God (the heavenly parent). The Bible is clear that the dead are without understanding (Ecclesiastes 9:5) and that worship offered to created beings is not God's way (Acts 10:25, 26; Revelation 19:10); hence, it is inappropriate to pray to and worship the dead. We are to acknowledge God as the ultimate source of life and worship Him, not our parents. Christians have no need to mourn as those without hope, for we look for the coming of the Lord in heaven. After the funeral, respect for departed loved ones most certainly can be shown by cleaning and caring for the grave and remembering them in fondness at the usual cultural times of remembrance. A special song of thanksgiving may be offered to God for the lives of parents at these times of remembrance. Participants can rededicate their lives to the heavenly parent.[438]

Religious rituals maintain family cohesion and commitment and give high value to family life with emphasis on love, respect, understanding, and forgiveness.

> *Religious rituals maintain family cohesion and commitment and give high value to family life*

There is a grand spiritual tradition that was introduced by God at the end of His creation of the world and the creatures in it. This tradition calls for the setting of a specific day of the week aside in which to acknowledge God (Saturday in today's world) as the superior ruling being in the universe (Deuteronomy 5:12–14). Such a practice also accepts His loving commitment to the welfare and salvation of the race. Such understandings are the basis for worship and explain the Christian's attitude and commitment to their creator. A philosophy based on the principles of love, loyalty, and commitment is incompatible with the exclusive pursuit of individual interests in a materialistic world devoid of hope. In consequence, the Christian is thankful, joyful, and positive (Psalm 63:5; Colossians 1:9–12). Perhaps not surprisingly, researchers have found that grateful individuals have a higher index of psychological and physical well-being than others.[439] Of course, an attitude of gratitude should not be restricted to a single day.

The moral and spiritual values that enable these positive outcomes to flourish are taken on more successfully in warm, loving families. Parents who are positive—accepting parents rather than cold, rejecting ones—are the most effective in transmitting moral values to their offspring. The other important aspect of parenting style is that those warm parents who administer punishment immediately and consistently are more effective in promoting knowledge of moral boundaries, especially if explanation accompanies the punishment. It is important for children to understand why an action is considered wrong. When children understand, they develop internal controls. Wise parents do not withdraw their love and do not use forceful language or other activities that generate anxiety, fear, and resentment. The children in such households take on the values not through fear and anxiety but because such behavior may "violate my positive self-image" or make me "feel guilty" or induce the comment "I'm feeling ashamed."[440] This taking on of values on account of internal discomfit rather than on account of external threats is exactly what the Bible instructs parents to achieve. The language is a little quaint but says that those approved of God "obeyed from the heart [or mind]." In other words, they first unreservedly accept God's values in principle and then put them into practice (Romans 6:17).

Highlights:

1. *Religious and spiritual rituals within a community of caring individuals allow family cohesion to be maintained effectively.*

2. *Traditions based on Christian values bring hope, optimism, and joy.*

3. *Moral and spiritual values are transmitted effectively in warm, loving families where an explanatory management style is the norm.*

Ideal Family Structures

The ideal family structure promoted will depend on the cultural and philosophical positions taken. For example, if the idea is embraced that life arose through random events and that the fittest alone survived throughout evolutionary history, then it makes sense to believe that the strategy adopted to ensure the survival of one's genes would undoubtedly involve the selection of many sexual partners in order to achieve this goal. Some cultural or religious considerations might also lead to polygamous relationships.[441] On the other hand, if the understanding is that God created the first human pair for harmonious, social relationships, with the purpose of reflecting His character, caring for the world, and populating it rationally so as to develop and protect its resources, then the model adopted would argue for one partner, heterosexual, and a same faith relationship (Genesis 2:20–24). This latter pattern of behavior was rejected at an early time as people chose to forget their origins and purpose. Polygamy became popular (Genesis 6:2),[442] and even same-sex partnerships were developed (Romans 1:24–32). In recent times, same-sex partnerships have been plagued by devastating disease outbreaks. If these were left to develop according to natural outcomes, in the absence of medical science, an incredible number of individuals would be eliminated. The decline in the family ideal is assisted by alternative partner arrangements, which promote individual concerns over community concerns. In advanced societies, the nuclear (or now egalitarian) family is the arrangement that works the best. They are at the center of a well-functioning civil society.[443]

Highlight: Nuclear (or now egalitarian) families are at the heart of a well-functioning civil society as planned by the Creator.

Parenting Style

The development of competent children will be dependent largely on the parenting style adopted. The three most emphasized parenting styles are authoritarian, permissive, and authoritative (there is also the indifferent style). By far the most successful style is the authoritative style. Such parents give consistent guidance and are warm and affectionate, yet firm. Effective parents give reasons for boundaries and encourage their children to think and make sound decisions. They have a democratic style of management, which means they dialogue with their children and do not use harsh forms of punishment; their children tend to be competent and self-controlled. They are able to act independently and have good coping skills.[444]

Effective parents give reasons for boundaries and encourage their children to think and make sound decisions.

These approaches are highlighted in Scripture. The prophet Eli indulged in a permissive parenting style, which gave rise to tragic results. His sons were corrupt, working in the service of God for gain, but he did not restrain them. In consequence, God judged both Eli and his sons (1 Samuel 3:10–14, 4:11, 17, 18). King Saul, on the other hand, was authoritarian and rash in his approach. This brought him into disgrace before his army (1 Samuel 14:24–30, 43–45). The advice of Scripture is to teach children right ways (authoritative rather than indifferent) and to avoid breaking their spirit (Deuteronomy 6:7–9; Proverbs 22:6; Ephesians 6:4). A brief glimpse into Mary and Joseph's household indicates that this was the parenting style they adopted with Jesus (Luke 2:42–52). In this approach, parents interact with their children who in turn learn from the experience.

Highlight: The authoritative parenting style is the most successful and is the one recommended in Scripture.

In practical terms, a successful authoritative style begins with forming an early mother/child bond and in speaking frequently and positively to children almost from birth. The approach, pioneered by Dr. Burton White, is summarized below. An important point to convey is that effective parenting is not dependent on modern, expensive toys or on the parents possessing university qualifications. The most relevant points in the early development of competent children are as follows:[445]

- Make the home safe and accessible to the child so that it can explore and investigate items of interest and common usage. Common items are provided for experimentation in an environment that does not endanger the child.

- Be available to give the child attention and support as required (responding to the cries of a child sympathetically develops trust). Prompt, favorable, and enthusiastic encouragement is healthy. Talk often and engage with children intellectually and emotionally and extend their vocabulary in easy steps.

- Talk often to the child and actively seek to understand their actions and what they see as significant. Expand their range of activities and words.

- Set limits to unacceptable behavior and requests. Do not spoil children.

- Provide new learning activities and allow them to assume responsibility for some of the shared activities as they grow. Encourage pretend activities, especially where adult roles are being attempted.

- Encourage spontaneous emotional responses.

Healthy functioning in families is dependent on developing clear forms of communication and effective problem solving, satisfying the emotional needs, showing genuine interest in the activities and interests of members, and supporting independent decisions and actions. Not surprisingly, communication patterns that convey impressions of support and warmth and engage in an explanatory and analytical style of communication are the most effective in giving children confidence in attempting to solve their own problems.[446]

Disciplinary issues are approached in the same manner. The reasons for requesting a particular course of action and the consequences of departures are explained. Such parents are the most likely to adopt moderate forms of discipline and respond as soon as departures are evident. Warm parents who administer punishments immediately and consistently are the most effective in promoting knowledge of moral boundaries, especially if explanation accompanies the punishment. This helps children to develop internal controls. Wise parents do not withdraw their love and do not use forceful language or other devices that generate anxiety, fear, and resentment. The children take on the values promoted, not through fear and anxiety, but through not wishing to feel ashamed and violating their own self-image.[447]

Highlight: A common sense approach to parenting delivers positive outcomes. This includes making the home safe, encouraging, and stimulating the child emotionally and intellectually, thus ensuring unacceptable behavior is understood and that the growing individual is taught to accept responsibility.

Guiding Principles and Practical Suggestions

1. Nuclear (or now egalitarian) families are at the heart of a well-functioning civil society as planned by the Creator. Family life is the place where moral values, worldview, social concerns, and creative approaches to life issues are developed.

2. A good parenting style can be learned and the benefits are measurable and continue well beyond preschool. The authoritative parenting style is the most successful and is the one recommended in Scripture.

3. Effective parents take clear stands on issues from the early years; they accept their authority roles.

4. Family background and attitudes have a major impact on achievement right through the school years. Parental interest and encouragement ensure that children gain the greatest benefit from their school experience.

5. In healthy families a wide range of feelings is expressed without the possibility of personal criticism or angry outbursts occurring. Comments are moderated and explanatory. There is genuine empathy among the members.

6. In well-adjusted families, decision-making power is shared. Parents are in control but aid the children in internalizing standards without recourse to authoritarian behavior.

7. Friendship networks help family members gain a better opinion of themselves and cope with the difficulties of parenting. The support of community members in transmitting moral values is highly significant. Moral values taught through the schooling system are successful in transmitting socially mature values to the young and aid in preventing the development of antisocial children.

8. Time provided together to communicate, make decisions, and enjoy each other's company is vital to healthy family functioning.

9. The strength of the bond between spouses is assessed in terms of ability to communicate, trust, love, and function in harmony. Emphasizing such characteristics provides for a strong family unit.

10. Religious and spiritual rituals are associated with healthy families. A belief system enables members to cope with loss within the supporting framework of a community of caring individuals.

11. Effective parenting is assisted by: making the home safe and accessible to the child; being available to give the child attention and support as required; setting limits to unacceptable behavior and requests; providing new learning activities; allowing them to assume responsibility for some of the shared activities as they grow; and encouraging spontaneous emotional responses.

12. Family involvement in community activities can be an ideal way in which to strengthen family bonds by working together to achieve group goals.

Chapter 9

Embracing Attractive Behaviors

Western societies have placed emphasis on personal independence, materialism, and success in contrast to some other societies. It should not be surprising that in Western societies success is seen as a reward for one's own efforts in fair competition with others, leading often to a self-centered approach to life. Some of those in managerial positions and occupations requiring specialized knowledge have flourished in our materialistic societies while others have been marginalized through a decline in the need for unskilled labor. Yet others are exposed to alienating conditions through an inability to have much control over their lives in the work environment. Those in the latter category have more stressful lives, and they reap the consequences in ill health.[448] Some argue that an emphasis on capitalism, selfish behavior,

and the like are simply an expression of our evolutionary inheritance and that the rise of individualism and lack of a closeness of community are a realization of our inborn tendencies. Naturally, there are competing views that see cooperation as a fundamental part of human nature.[449] I will look at some of these issues later in this chapter.

The pursuit of the good life often involves intense competition and uncertainty and can lead to nervous exhaustion and stress. Modern living is not conducive to enduring, close relationships with our fellow citizens, particularly as a majority of people live in large cities. These cities, by their very nature, do not make some forms of networking easy with a wide group of friends with different interests and perspectives. It is also difficult to form close, enduring friendships. Even more difficult is the idea of working for the common good where the overwhelming sentiment is to further one's private interest by hard work and initiative. Understandably, civic pride and participation in community activities for the betterment of all can be more commonly experienced in small communities.[450]

Finding a way to reclaim the sense of community can be achieved in large population centers.

However, finding a way to reclaim the sense of community can be achieved in large population centers. Religious groups, particularly Christians, are well able to develop a common bond among believers that can be expressed in practical love and acceptance. This experience may change a person's view of marriage, work associates, and the world. Others immerse themselves in groups with common interests in ethnic, environmental, and political affairs that give them a sense of being part of a community, even of the world community.[451] This sense of community can be a significant contributor to the way in which we behave. For example, the notable whistleblowers (Coleen Rowley—FBI, Cynthia Cooper—WorldCom, and Sherron Watkins—Enron), nominated 2002 Persons of the Year, believed "that where they worked was a place that served a wider world in some important way."[452]

Those committed to community interests may show the following features:[453]

- Long-term commitments are made based on the idea of investment in the future. Fleeting feelings are not the basis of actions.

- Freedom of action is based on values shared and modeled by others. These values are derived from ideals of character and do not lead to the denial of well-defined commitments already made by the individual.

- Civic action is based on an understanding that upholding universally acceptable values fulfills personal identity. An appreciation for the dignity of individuals and their susceptibility to the abuse of power leads to identification with them because these values have universal acceptance.[454]

- Social involvement is a form of self-determination that strengthens the individual to resist conformity and to develop resilience.

Highlight: Civic pride and a sense of community responsibility are promoted by Christian congregations and progressive elements in society and represent commitments made from high ideals.

In the following section, I wish to explore briefly some understandings that promote the development of social responsibility.

Perspectives on Social Responsibility

Concepts of social responsibility in the family, community, and the world community ultimately derive from the philosophy accepted to describe reality. Those developed in the ancient Christian scriptures have modern relevance, and I will develop these more fully in a future chapter dealing with the questions of being and the nature of humans. Suffice it to say here that ideas nurtured to explain the nature of humanity influence thinking on human purpose and equity. These views ultimately impact on our understandings of the dignity of the human race and of individuals and thus on social responsibility.

Human Dignity

All human beings are entitled to respect irrespective of age, sex, ethnic origin, health status, and social or religious affiliations simply owing to the fact that they are members of the human race. Humans enjoy a common origin. If one accepts the idea of a singular creation event, as explained in the Christian scriptures, all then are equal by creation. They are of "one blood" as the physician Luke tells us succinctly (Acts 17:26). The concept of equality is strengthened in this communion by the argument that each member of the human race has been bought by the death of Christ.

The death of Christ, at infinite cost, has established each individual as being of great worth.

The death of Christ, at infinite cost, has established each individual as being of great worth (John 3:16; Luke 23:39–43; John 4:9, 10).[455] The Christian humbly acknowledges this and recognizes that the only response possible is to accept the love offered (1 John 3:1–3). In consequence, believers have a firm self-respect, but arrogant pride and self-importance do not form part of their developing self-image. They are happy to be called followers of Christ and are delighted to reflect His noble principles to others. As a consequence, they show strength of character that is evident to all.[456]

Highlight: *Humans are of a common origin, and each individual has been given infinite value by the death of Christ. This confers dignity on all.*

Philosophical Base

The duty of parents is to help children develop a balanced view of their origin, destiny, abilities, opportunities, values, and responsibilities. Loving, accepting, and involved parents, who have a democratic parenting style and who get along well, assist the development of a realistic concept of the children's potential and dignity as individuals.[457] Prosocial behavior (promotes social acceptance and friendship), not surprisingly, is also linked to the values accepted.

Societies or subgroups within society that foster cooperative behavior and responsibility are more likely to produce children who are anxious about others. The values accepted by the Christian ideally make prosocial behavior a way of thinking. This is based on the understandings that God created humans as social beings, has given people their inherent skills, and has paid the ransom price for the salvation of each member of the human family (Deuteronomy 8:18; Psalm 24:1; Romans 5:8). As a result, both small as well as large commitments are made to the well-being of others (Exodus 32:32–34; Matthew 25:37–40). Concern begins in the neighborhood and stretches globally. There can be no greater realization that the individual is indebted to humanity than the joyful, experiential knowledge of salvation and the assurance from Scripture that the believing individual is God's representative (Matthew 28:19, 20; 2 Corinthians 5:20). Systematic benevolence is a natural response to these understandings (Malachi 3:8). Such a commitment is bound to change priorities and strengthen the resolve of individuals to be involved in prosocial activities.

On the other hand, aggressive or antisocial behavior is also linked to the norms and values accepted in the subcultures in which a person is operating. This is only part of the picture, but there are some societies that are antisocial on account of ideas of independence and combativeness and emotional unresponsiveness taught and valued by these groups.[458]

Highlights:

1. *Prosocial behavior is part of the response anticipated as coming from born-again Christians.*

2. *Prosocial behavior is linked to the values accepted and taught.*

The question I will address in the following section is how ideas of social responsibility are transmitted.

Learning to Benefit Others

An important question that we might well ask is: How do children gain the desire to participate in community and public involvement or become committed to prosocial behavior? Certainly, a lack of social involvement in times of crisis can have tragic consequences as the murder of Kitty Genovese in 1964 brought home to many. Retiring home late at night she was attacked and repeatedly stabbed and finally died after alerting neighbors by her screaming. Not one of the thirty-eight neighbors watching called the police.[459] By contrast, selfless acts of heroism (altruism) are applauded by society. Awards, medals, and ceremonies accompany such recognition. Unapplauded, but highly appreciated, are the hundreds of people who donate an organ to another person.[460]

In the search for an answer to our question, we will not be particularly interested in the fine distinctions made regarding motivations for helping, sharing, and comforting. It is undeniable that some acts rebound on the giver in positive outcomes. Indeed, reinforcing positive behaviors are at the foundation of favoring socially responsible (prosocial) attitudes, whether given by parents or peer models.[461]

Parental Attitudes

The roots of prosocial behavior are sown early—in the toddler phase of development. It has been found that less compassionate toddlers have mothers who are more prone to deliver physical restraint or punishment and restrict behavior without explanation. Explaining the connection between acts and their effects on others is important in the early training of children. The behavior acquired during childhood appears to be fairly stable. As children age they also become more discriminating and analyze the reasons for a person's misfortune before they offer help.[462] There is a strong relationship between the development of prosocial behavior in children and warm, loving parents who principally discipline by explanation followed by non-punitive measures.[463] This is a good model to adopt and is also the biblical advice (1 Samuel 1:20–28; 2:18–20, 26; Ephesians 6:4).

Less compassionate toddlers have mothers who are more prone to deliver physical restraint or punishment and restrict behavior without explanation.

The development of prosocial behavior can be aided by activities that help children recognize what others are feeling, thinking, or aiming to achieve. Moral reasoning makes important contributions to the ability of teenagers to respond to the needs and wishes of others. When a person can experience the emotions of others (empathy), it becomes easier to participate in prosocial behavior.[464] Prosocial behavior is initiated in the family and the interacting society aids in this endeavor. The influences in our families and society that particularly encourage prosocial behavior are as follows:[465]

- Develop family structures that encourage contributions to the welfare of the group through the activities of all members.

- Balance ideas of competition and individual goals with group goals and interests.

- Promote socially responsible behavior through verbal approval rather than through giving material rewards.

- Develop a genuine warm relationship with children so that praise given for their socially responsible attitudes is reinforced.

- Develop a parenting style that relies on explanations and less forceful ways of correcting wrongdoing.

- Play cooperative games to achieve easily defined goals rather than games that are based on individual activities.

- Practice what you say. Positive modeling of activities helpful to others will contribute to children and young people accepting the principles. On the other hand, refusal to follow through your own advice will lead to a poor result.

- Avoid exposure to aggressive toys, games, and television images.

Individuals who have active concern for others are able to enter into their feelings. We say that such individuals have acquired moral knowledge, which they use to inform their judgments. They tend to be honest, dedicated to tasks, and given to self-control.[466]

The family is the institution that has a significant influence on the development of social and community values. The nuclear (or now egalitarian) family is the best structure available in the Western world to transmit such values. In the East there is a greater emphasis on family group participation in contrast to the West. Western structures tend to foster individualism. They may fair badly in teaching prosocial behavior, for they often foster individual interests and reward the competitive in the achievement of personal goals. Sharing may not be high on the agenda.[467] Such behaviors do not provide a good model for others and indicate the need for a stronger philosophical base to underpin the educational process.

Society is dependent upon the family to develop civic values in children so that they show honesty, trust, self-sacrifice, and personal responsibility. These values must be taught early in life. In families where there is an extreme emphasis on individual interests of the members, selfish behavior is strengthened and the concerns of society minimized. This contributes to the fragmentation of society.[468]

Positive modeling of behavior is highly significant.

Positive modeling of behavior is highly significant. The models used may be parental or non-parental. Studies have shown that children who possess positive role models have higher self-esteem, higher grades, a stronger sense of identity, and are more likely to avoid participating in negative behaviors than those who lack role models. It appears that gender matched models have a greater impact than when models are not matched (i.e., adolescent females have female role models, etc.). It is commonly observed that parental models are most influential in the life of adolescents, for they are the people with whom adolescents have regular contact. The tendency is for adolescent females to look to their mothers and males to look to their fathers for guidance. Having several role models strengthened the positive outcomes.[469]

Those who practice positive modeling understand that what is said must be practiced if we wish to make a favorable impact (Matthew 23:1–4). Promises without corresponding deeds do little to foster prosocial behavior among humans and have no value in God's sight. We should be especially careful to live what we believe and fulfill promises made. For example, parents' lack of concern and cold relationships with their children will ultimately be mirrored in the behavior of their children. Indifference about the whereabouts of adolescents and their activities also contributes to aggression, similar to conflict between the adults in the family setting.[470] The examples left for Christians to consider and follow in the Scriptures are substantial. God's promise (and its ultimate fulfillment) to send the Savior is a magnificent display of social responsibility. This promise was fulfilled in a spectacular fashion in the life and death of Christ on earth and His subsequent ministry in heaven (Genesis 3:15; Ecclesiastes 5:4–7; John 3:16; Hebrews 7:24–27; 8:1–6).

Alternatively, aggressive modeling and non-cooperative behavior will have an adverse effect on values. Such behavior often is featured on television and in video and computer games and this form of entertainment can instruct in antisocial and criminal behavior. Careful selection of programs showing friendliness, self-control, and prosocial activities can strengthen the beneficial outcomes. Exposure to aggressive TV shows and violent video games in early childhood is particularly damaging.[471] A Christian should especially act honorably when tempted to think and meditate (and particularly looking in our day and age) on impure, lying, and aggressive activities (Psalm 101:3; Philippians 4:8). The informed Christian attitude is to repudiate trends in society that glorify aggression, violence, unfaithfulness, lust, riotous, rude, unloving, and uncaring behavior. Christian parents seek to provide moral insights, a supportive social environment, training in civilized behavior, and service to others within a holistic and purposeful framework. In

this respect, there is much in common with the Muslim position.[472]

Highlights:

1. *Socially responsible behavior is taught first in the family through leading the young to enter into the feelings of others by explanation and active involvement.*

2. *Involvement in cooperative activities is most effective when mentors practice the principles taught and develop warm relationships with those they are mentoring.*

3. *Exposure to non-cooperative games and aggressive activities lead to poor outcomes, especially where mentors are cold and resort to physical punishment.*

Moral Values

The practices adopted by the supporting community are relevant in encouraging prosocial behavior. Even atheistic regimes have understood the value of moral training. When stress is placed on prosocial behavior (sharing, collective play, and work activities) and consideration and self-discipline, the children going through such experiences take on the values taught. Perhaps surprisingly, the former Soviet Union produced children in the 1960s and 1970s with fewer tendencies to antisocial behavior than their counterparts in the United States (a Christian nation). Public schools in the latter country took the attitude that it was not their job to teach moral values, an attitude derived no doubt from the idea that moral values are relative rather than absolute and that the state has no rights in the business of moral education.[473] One publicized experiment on a national scale, where the ideas of Nietzsche (who advocated relative values) were put into practice, was in Nazi Germany. In a speech Adolf Hitler said: "I desire to create a generation without conscience, imperious, relentless, and cruel."[474]

He was observably successful and he destroyed his nation. Every nation deserves a better outcome; hence, a firmer foundation of responsibility than relative values must be diligently sought if national greatness is valued.

The former Soviet Union produced children... with fewer tendencies to antisocial behavior than their counterparts in the United States

---

Moral values such as diligence, honesty, economy, discipline, politeness, hygiene, harmony, and generosity need to be taught in a systematic fashion. This is understood clearly within the Kingdom of Thailand, which is a Buddhist nation. The National Education Act specifies that all aspects of morality should be taught and that this is an effort that involves families, communities, religious, and educational institutions.[475] In many Western nations, the trend has been to distance training in character development and civic responsibilities from religious affiliation and to emphasize shared cultural values.[476]

Christian education has gone through its own substantial changes, but exists on account of the concern to effectively transmit moral values and other core values such as character development, relationships, and service to others. Such values are based on virtues illustrated in the lives of the individuals highlighted in the Bible's pages and on principles enunciated there. A basic belief is that morality has a Judeo-Christian foundation, ultimately based on divine revelation. This means that, to varying degrees in Christian schools,

character education is associated with emphasis on ritual and liturgical aspects of the faith.[477]

The reality is that surrounding children with dedicated and committed role models during their formative years is the best guarantee that they will internalize the values upheld. One of the strong beliefs in the Christian community is that moral values came directly to humanity as a result of divine revelation (Exodus 20:1–17; 31:18). These principles are summarized in the Decalogue (Ten Commandments) and represent to believers something that is unalterable and universally applicable. In other words, they represent the gold standard for all moral thinking. Indeed, many of these principles are incorporated into other belief systems that arose after the time God delivered His moral road map. Ethical standards accepted in the world today also trace their roots to this code.[478]

Highlights:

1. *Moral values can be taught effectively in a systematic fashion in the educational system.*

2. *Christian communities are well suited to teach moral values based on the principles of the Decalogue.*

Guiding Principles and Practical Suggestions

1. The sense of community and cooperation is rooted in the meta-narrative or worldview adopted.

2. Community interests are more fully evident in individuals who make long-term commitments and thus invest in the future; they adopt values derived from ideals of character (with universal acceptance) and believe that upholding such values fulfills personal identity; they believe that social involvement is a form of self-determination that strengthens the individual to resist conformity and to be resilient.

3. The foundations of prosocial behavior are sown early (toddler phase of development).

4. Reinforcing positive behaviors are at the foundation of favoring socially responsible (prosocial) attitudes. Such behavior can be aided by activities that help children recognize what others are feeling, thinking or aiming to achieve.

5. Moral reasoning makes important contributions to the ability of children and teenagers to respond to the needs and wishes of others.

6. Experiencing the emotions of others (empathy) makes it easier to participate in prosocial behavior.

7. Prosocial behavior is associated with activities that encourage contributions to the welfare of the group through the activities of all members and balance ideas of competition and individual goals with group goals and interests.

8. Socially responsible behavior is best developed through warm verbal approval rather than through giving material rewards. Explanatory parenting styles are more effective than forceful ways to correct wrongdoing.

9. Positive modeling of activities helpful to others will contribute to children and young people accepting the principles.

10. Exposure to aggressive toys, games, and television images fails to promote prosocial behavior and contributes to the destruction of society.

11. Moral values are transmitted effectively as family, community, religious, and educational institutions combine their efforts.

12. Moral values of universal applicability, which will protect every society, are found in the Decalogue. Moral values established through consensus are not acceptable to Christians.

Chapter 10

Escaping From Mayhem

Stress is a part of our lives. In our attempts to adapt to the changing environment we find ourselves in and raise families in a challenging world, it is inevitable that we will experience stress at some point. Coping with this is critical to the health of each individual and their families. In order to maintain emotional and social stability, individuals must be able to cope with stress. Each individual must appraise the effects that changes to their environment will make and whether these are likely to be a threat. If personal well-being is threatened by the changing circumstances, then the individual will react emotionally. The level of stress will be moderated by the coping resources that the individual believes are available. This means that situations will impact each person differently.[479]

Understanding a few details about the sequence of physiologic events associated with stressful experiences will aid the discussion. If the body is in a state of arousal (under threat), the levels of flight or fight hormone or messenger molecules coming from the adrenal glands are elevated, i.e., catecholamine levels—adrenaline (epinephrine) and norepinephrine. A response is seen ultimately in the elevation of the heart rate, blood pressure, and blood glucose levels. The response prepares the body for muscular activity. Once the threat is removed, the body returns to normal. A longer lasting response to stress is provided by another group of adrenal hormones—corticosteroids of which cortisol is the most significant. Cortisol increases blood glucose concentrations at the expense of protein and fatty acid reserves. Where the response strategy of the individual is passive (as in coping with psychosocial stress) rather than active (as in escaping physical injury), corticosteroid hormone levels may be elevated unrealistically. When stress hormone levels (e.g., epinephrine and corticosteroids) remain elevated, it is thought that problems such as high blood pressure begin to develop. Issues arise as the resources made available to the body are not used. In addition, there is a prolonged exposure to stress hormones, which at certain levels have deleterious effects particularly on the immune system.[480]

Stress is important to us because it ultimately affects our health. The elevated hormone levels may render the individual more susceptible to hypertension and other diseases.[481] Hypertension is a blood vessel disease—hardening of the arteries. This is not a simple condition but is influenced by heredity and diet together with stress. In hardening of the arteries, fatty deposits (LDLs) form in the interior of the arteries (and eventually a lesion protrudes into the opening of the vessel). Now this process of depositing fatty acids is accelerated when the blood pressure is elevated—exactly the condition created by stress. Vigorous exercise performed at the same time as the fatty acid levels are raised leads to their clearance from the system, but if this does not occur they are deposited on the artery walls.[482]

Other factors complicate the scene. For example, in the investigation of personality, various types have been identified. Individuals with type A behavior are understood perhaps more than the other type. Such individuals are very competitive, tend to be in a hurry, are active on many projects and are prone to hostility—they tend to be more stress prone. The last emotional characteristic, if not controlled, is a good indicator of coronary heart disease. For this type of individual, some change in behavior is warranted if long life is desired.[483]

A range of gastrointestinal problems also are associated with psychological distress.[484] Of particular interest is the formation of stress ulcers of the stomach. It is suggested that on account of stress, blood flow is reduced and thus the flow of nutrients and oxygen to the stomach is correspondingly reduced. Oxygen and nutrients are needed to make sure that the stomach wall and its protective mucus covering are maintained. When these nutrients are not supplied in normal amounts, then there is some deficit in maintaining a healthy stomach wall due to shortcomings in the production of protective chemicals, leaving the wall exposed to the corroding effects of the acid gastric juices. It is at the end of the period of the stress where the damage is done, for the stomach wall is not fully protected on the resumption of acid production.[485]

Stress has some impact on the immune system too and, therefore, the ability of the body to combat disease. The exact nature of these effects is not known, but those with effective coping strategies are in a better condition to maintain immune system function. An interesting link also has been suggested between stress and the ability of the animal body to control the growth of certain tumors. The relationship between psychosocial stress, hormone levels, and cancer growth in humans has still to be established firmly, but it is an area of interest and research. Then there is increasing evidence of an interrelationship between stress and the onset or progression of chronic diseases. The nervous system interacts with the endocrine and immune system in complex ways.[486] In future years these complex interactions will be understood more clearly.

Another interesting link, that some are not anxious to talk about, is the one between human spirituality and stress. This relationship is so strong that the scientific world speaks convincingly of the impact of religious involvement on physical and emotional health.[487] I will deal with spirituality in another chapter, but first I will look at strategies of coping with stress.

Highlight: Unrelieved stress can render an individual more prone to blood vessel disease, gastro-intestinal problems and more susceptible to disease organisms through suboptimal functioning of the immune system.

Coping Strategies to Minimize Stress

When we are faced with stresses, coping strategies are put into place. We will not consider, beyond a brief mention, such coping strategies as taking drugs, overeating, and the like. These are destructive strategies; it is our intention to focus on constructive ideas. Such strategies may be put in place almost unconsciously but, if the stress is continuous and complex, a more directed approach is necessary. Positive and successful problem-focused approaches to coping possess four components:[488]

- Increase awareness. Focus on the nature of the problem from a range of perspectives; do not be satisfied with the current narrow view.

- Process information. Explore ways to change the stressful sensory inputs. Look at the options and resources available.

- Investigate avenues for behavior modification. Explore peaceful avenues of resolving the problem that may include new actions and modified behaviors.

- Peaceful resolution. Resolve the problem peacefully so that satisfactory relationships with others can be maintained.

The ability to resolve stressful situations peacefully through taking risks and seeking new pathways of action is easier for some personality types than for others. However, there are many strategies available, and the good news is that coping skills increase with practice. First, the individual must be willing to take an active role in resolving stress. Secondly, both the body and mind must be intimately involved in stress management. Sometimes it is useful to disengage mentally from a stressful situation and become distracted with other issues. However, this does not represent a useful long-term solution to the problem. In the long-term such strategies become dysfunctional and counterproductive.[489]

Highlight: Stress may be reduced through adopting a directed and creative approach to the problem.

Strategies to reduce stress have been put into various categories. Often these are spoken about as problem-focused and emotion-focused. The former is where reduction or removal of the stressor is sought and the latter relates to efforts to reduce or minimize emotional consequences. There are other ways of looking at coping. Avoidance coping represents a disengagement from the issues experienced, but it confers minimal advantages beyond the immediate situation. However, the reality is that coping strategies may not fit easily into these categories. Adaptive responses often complement each other—emotional relief often comes from problem solving sessions and *vice versa*.[490] The individual will choose from among these to suit their purpose.

I will briefly mention some of the skills that are thought primarily as coping devices.[491]

Attitude Adjustment

This is a process of accepting responsibility and expanding the field of possible solutions rather than restricting them. The successful individual is optimistic about the resolution of the problem.

Coping with stress effectively involves taking responsibility rather than trying to shift it somewhere else, searching for excuses or blaming others. The effective person takes a positive (optimistic) attitude and searches for solutions and even tries to find something worthwhile in the situation by looking at the problem from a different viewpoint. The movement is away from ideas of victimization, in order to bathe in the sympathy of others, to a positive approach to life. We need to make the most of a situation, not the worst by blowing things out of proportion. After all, our health will be influenced by our attitudes.[492]

> *Coping with stress effectively involves taking responsibility rather than trying to shift it somewhere else.*

One interesting story that comes to us from antiquity pictures the progenitors of the human race being persuaded by Satan into disobeying their divine Maker. The man, who followed the woman's example of disobedience, blamed her and her maker (God) for the poor results that followed their course of action, and the woman, who was deceived, blamed the agent through whom the deceiver spoke (Genesis 3:11–13). Ultimately, they were trying to avoid direct responsibility for their actions. This story comes down to us in ancient manuscripts to warn us of the unsatisfactory consequences of not accepting responsibility for our own actions.

There is another famous story that tells us that optimism is likely to win the day. This story is set in the time of Joshua, in the ancient history of Israel, when twelve spies were sent to the land in the vicinity of Jerusalem to assist in planning its conquest in the near future. Ten of the spies saw only the difficulties; only two saw the possibilities. The majority of the spies told such a convincing story that most of the people believed them and became

very disappointed and even aggressive against those who expressed confidence in the success of the battle plans (Numbers 13:27–31; 14:1–10). The attitude the majority displayed was a self-fulfilling prophecy, so much so that they did not succeed in their conquest attempt a short time later (Numbers 14:35–45). However, after forty years, when optimism was the watchword, success was achieved (Joshua 5, 6).

Tough situations may cause shock and depression. These are not regarded as harmful as long as the individual can move on, within a reasonable period of time, to more productive areas of thought and action. In instances where it is impossible to change a situation, acceptance in a spirit of serenity is highly beneficial.[493] Of course, the Christian argues strenuously that God is able to help achieve such an attitude of serenity (2 Corinthians 12:7–10). The episode recorded by the apostle Paul indicates that it is how we relate to the situations we find ourselves in that is important.

Highlight: Taking responsibility for a situation and being optimistic about the future are good approaches to relieving stress.

Behavior Modification

Changing one behavioral pattern for another option involves awareness, a desire to change, and then conscious choice at the point of action to substitute a more appropriate alternative. This may involve a willingness to express one's feelings (assertive) without being either passive or aggressive.

The remarkable change in the behavior of Peter, one of the founding apostles of the Christian church, is well recorded by historical sources and constitutes a good example of behavior modification (Matthew 26:74, 75; Acts 4:13). The change was from a cursing, cowering fisherman to an eloquent, confident public speaker and evangelist. When threatened by his hearers, Peter replied in confident (assertive) fashion (Acts 4:18–20). This same Peter went on to serve his Lord honorably and died by crucifixion (John 21:18, 19). If it had been possible to measure the health benefits flowing from such changes, they probably would have been remarkable, as witnessed by scientists in related situations today.[494]

In order to change behavior, we must first be aware of our undesirable characteristics and wish to change. With this heightened awareness, at the moment when an action is about to be initiated, the new direction can be brought into focus. This new course of action is put into place, improvements are noted, and desirable further refinements devised.[495] For the Christian, the process is the same except for the important difference that the person asks for God's help in making such changes. At the point of temptation or desired change, we can ask for divine help with confidence, knowing that it will be given (Romans 6:5, 6; 1 Corinthians 10:13).

The values we adopt in life influence our attitude and the behaviors we seek to see developed. The story of Joseph, whose adult life began as a slave and ended as a state official (Genesis 39:7–20; 41:37–43),[496] is worth noticing. His behavior was derived from his attitude toward God that in turn was based on principle. The principle that he acted upon is clearly stated in the moral code adopted by Christians. As a consequence, he rejected self-serving behavior, which was ultimately the secret of his success (Exodus 20:14).

If we are to change our behavior then our attitudes, and ultimately our principles of action, must be rethought.

It stands to reason that if we are to change our behavior then our attitudes, and ultimately our principles of action, must be rethought. The Christian is fortunate in that a moral code, which has stood the test of time, is readily accessible. I will look at this set of values in a subsequent chapter.

Highlight: *Awareness of better alternatives, a desire to change, and deliberate choice at the critical time are steps designed to promote changes in behavior.*

Creative Problem Solving

Creative problem solving is the art of finding new ways of approaching problems rather than believing there is only one way something can be done and that others have all the answers. The secret is to tease out the components of a larger problem into smaller, distinct issues. Multiple solutions are then imagined, and finally, the pros and cons of adopting these are considered. An option is selected on the basis of the analysis and it is implemented and finally evaluated. If the problem is not resolved, then the process is repeated on the basis of the greater knowledge acquired.[497]

Sometimes in the Christian church it is considered that there is only one right way in which to do things because that is the manner it has been done traditionally. However, this may not be the appropriate manner to find a workable solution. In the early Christian church, an intense dispute developed between Paul and Barnabas about the inclusion of John Mark in an evangelistic team (Acts 15:36–40). The problem apparently arose because each thought their way of doing things was correct. There are usually many ways of solving problems, especially when moral or ethical issues are not involved. Making order out of chaos requires creative thinking. Those who can think outside the square and find different ways of doing things can come up with a game plan that can potentially end in resolution of the issue being considered. This functions to reduce stress. Creative problem solving is one of the most important coping skills.[498]

Some of the most brilliant examples of creative problem solving in the Bible relate to the life of Jesus. He showed by example that resolution need not be a long and complicated process (Matthew 22:15–22; John 8:4–11).

Highlight: Creative problem solving, or thinking outside the box, is an important coping skill.

Communication Skills

All relationships are dependent upon communication that involves both self-disclosure and listening. Conflicts may arise when poor communication occurs. The most effective ways in which conflict can be resolved is through the use of persuasion and dialogue.

In contrast to our last story about Paul and Barnabas, where conflict was evident, the first church council held in Jerusalem had a happy ending because the people involved communicated effectively (Acts 15:1–21). It has been said that the three most important things to bring to a relationship are communication, communication, and communication. In the account recorded in our text, the individuals were involved in a dialogue style of conflict resolution where opinions and facts were exchanged frankly. A compromise position[499]—that did not neglect principle—was adopted. For the Christian, communication with God is equally significant. We are advised to "pray without ceasing" (1 Thessalonians 5:17) or, in other words, communicate, communicate, and communicate with God throughout the day.

An important therapeutic activity to assist with stress relief is simply the act of admitting our faults and blunders and putting things right as far as we are able (James 5:16). We are assured by the apostle James that disclosure of feelings lightens one's stress and leaves the individual in a frame of mind better able to enter into the healing prayer of faith. We need to put things right with our fellow men and then confess our shortcomings to God

and Him alone. Happily, we do not need human mediators or priests for us to gain access to God (1 Timothy 2:5; 1 John 1:9).

Highlight: Frank disclosure, putting things right, and listening are important aspects of communication that can function to relieve stress.

Time Management

The management of time, so that tasks are prioritized, scheduled, and executed, is a skill that can be learned. The importance of balancing work and play (personal time) is a neglected ingredient in the lives of some. An excessive workload is not abnormal in the day in which we live. This may be experienced by a wide cross section of people. For leaders there is a possible solution, as illustrated by an excellent example from an ancient story recorded by the historian Josephus.[500]

Moses, the prophet, who was designated by God to lead a vast group of slaves from Egypt to Israel, quite naturally experienced an excessive workload. His father-in-law (Jethro) suggested that delegation of authority would be a sensible alternative. It was an effective method to relieve the stress in one area of leadership undertaken by Moses. The general technique adopted by Jethro was one of analysis of the situation, laying out the options, and choosing the one giving the best solution to the problem (Exodus 18:13–24). The ideas of prioritization, organizing time segments to these priorities, and then putting the plan into operation can perhaps be seen in this biblical account.[501]

Sometimes tasks cannot be delegated to others and people attempt to multitask. This is the practice of trying to do two tasks at once (reading an e-mail and listening to a phone conversation) or switching rapidly among a group of tasks rather than completing the task (or a designated portion—chunk) before moving onto the next. Whereas some proclaim multitasking as a great method of moving through a mountain of work and pride themselves on their efficiency, this opinion is changing. If we take airline pilots as an example, multitasking has been found to contribute to the large number of dangerous incidents experienced on runways. Danger also lurks when we try to do several things while driving a car. In other situations, less is accomplished when attention is interrupted continually. The brain must refocus. Productivity goes down significantly and more errors are made. Stress levels also rise and interpersonal relationships suffer. More sensible approaches need to be put in place rather than adopting a multitask strategy.[502]

The work environment defines the existence of many people at higher levels of responsibility and management. The effort invested is justified in terms of immediate or short-term observable returns. In contrast, investment in the family takes many years to realize and lack of investment in health can take even longer. The challenge is to break out of the mindset that has trapped so many and give time to the things and people that really matter. Daniel Petre, the author of our resource reference, was one high profile manager who had the courage to change jobs in an attempt to get off the corporate treadmill so that he could spend time with his family and others who were valuable to him.[503] This is obviously one coping strategy that requires real courage.

Jesus' example is worth emulating. He gave Himself time to meditate, relax, and pray.

Personal time relates to time devoted to personal development. For the Christian, Jesus' example is worth emulating. He gave Himself time to meditate, relax, and pray (Matthew 14:23). We also find that He practiced a day of complete rest that in the Scriptures is called the Sabbath (Saturday), which was made by God for the benefit and enjoyment of humans (Mark 2:27; Luke 4:16).

Highlights:

1. *Prioritization, scheduling, and executing tasks are well tested coping skills.*
2. *Time set aside for personal and spiritual development will benefit health.*

There are a number of other coping devices that merit some comment. These have a strong emotional component, but they can assist in resolving issues.

Catharsis

This represents the process of relating a painful experience to a trusted individual rather than keeping the event secret. Even writing this experience down, so as to express the deepest thoughts and emotions, may have a positive effect on the health of the individual, as judged by improvement to immune system functioning and reduced consultations with doctors.[504] Perhaps a good Bible example of catharsis comes from the experience of Jonah. He was at first rather secretive about disobeying God and tried to avoid his assigned task by taking a boat to a foreign country. A violent storm arose, but he avoided the company of the sailors who were battling to keep the ship afloat. When finally he was accosted by the captain, he related to the ship's crew the nature of his shameful experience. It was only then that he felt better about accepting the consequences. He actually convinced the sailors to throw him into the sea in the belief that the wrath of God would be modified and the storm would subside. He survived the experience and went on to fulfill God's will (Jonah 1:5–17; 2:10; 3:1–4).

Forgiveness

Festering anger only leads to harm (Psalm 37:8). Avoidance of issues is not the answer to stress, but forgiveness is. Scripture gives the sound advice to get one's anger under control within the day (Ephesians 4:26). It was Albert Einstein who said, "Anger dwells only in the bosom of fools."[505] Perhaps to our surprise, forgiveness is considered a serious coping device.

The advice is to move on from anger and forgive the person(s) who has been instrumental in causing negative feelings through their actions. Negative feelings lead to toxic thoughts, and this renders us vulnerable to stress and loss of self-respect. The advice is: Be a survivor, not a victim.[506]

Prayer

Another coping device is prayer. We might be inclined to dismiss prayer, but it is interesting to note that the relevant part of the scientific world understands that prayer gives hope and fosters optimism and functions to lower anxiety. In a study of coping strategies among nurses in Singapore, it is worthwhile noting that prayer was regularly used by around 57 percent of respondents.[507]

How this might be used in the encounters of daily life comes from an episode captured in history from the kingdom of ancient Persia. Nehemiah, the royal cupbearer, was distressed at the news that his beloved Jerusalem was not being rebuilt. He developed a plan to introduce the problem to the king under favorable circumstances. However, his general expression of sadness made the king uncomfortable and he asked the reason for his mood change. Such expressions of distress might very well cause the king's displeasure and the offending servant could be punished. Nehemiah prayed for wisdom in this tense situation. He remained calm, as he stood before the king, and gained a favorable outcome (Nehemiah 2:2–5).

Others have used prayer similarly. Take Daniel the high court official in the kingdom of Babylon who served before Darius in the Medo-Persian Empire (Daniel 5:11–12; 6:1–3). Daniel is pictured in the historic account as still grappling with a stressful problem that caused him initially to faint and be sick (Daniel 8:27; 9:2–22). We find him again asking for divine help in prayer in order to understand the future prospects of the Jewish people and God's kingdom. His concerns were finally swept aside by a divine revelation in answer to his plea.

Highlight: Forgiveness and prayer are serious coping devices. Sharing hurts with sympathetic people (catharsis) is also useful in reducing stress.

More Emotionally Focused Approaches

Closely connected to the coping skills mentioned above are relaxation and other emotionally focused approaches that lessen distress. These techniques are aimed at mood regulation. They may do little to change the source of the stressful experience. Some relaxation techniques are humor therapy, music, art, meditation, and exercise. Social interaction and seeking life transformation through spiritual avenues may also lesson distress and give resilience. In fact, any device that operates to reduce distress and negative emotions can be considered under this heading. I will elaborate on several of these approaches.

Humor

Ancient cultures have regarded humor positively (Proverbs 17:22). An interesting biblical account, well known even to children, took place on Mount Carmel near to the modern city of Haifa where two guiding philosophies were in dispute and a showdown was imminent. The devise used to relieve tension was humor (1 Kings 18:27–29). This account sets the scene where Elijah was the sole representative of the creator-God. In contrast, there were many priests present who were devoted to the worship of Baal (god of the Phoenicians and Canaanites). The situation was extremely tense but, in a bold move, Elijah introduced exaggeration, as a form of humor, into dialogue. He asked the devotees of Baal to shout more loudly to awaken their god from slumber or other activities in order to focus his mind on his followers. They took the comments seriously. No doubt the device relieved the tension for Elijah as he observed their pointless activities.

Positive emotions can confer remarkable benefits on health.

The use of humor is one activity that is in the news. Positive emotions can confer remarkable benefits on health. The experience of Norman Cousins' remission and recovery from a rare rheumatoid disease, primarily through self-administered humor therapy, was vitally important in the emergence of the field of study known as psychoneuroimmunology. Today, humor is a well-attested coping strategy and relaxation technique that brings the body back to a balanced condition and maintains the functioning of the immune system. It is not a cure all, but it cannot be dismissed.[508]

Music

There is no serious question about the ability of music to rouse or soothe the emotions. Music is able to stimulate a variety of emotions of which relaxation is one. Dentists and physicians have introduced appropriate (instrumental music with a slow tempo) background music to their waiting areas in order to reduce client anxiety.[509] Music is thought primarily as a relaxation technique rather than a coping strategy.[510] The device actually has been used for many years.

An ancient account of music therapy comes from the experience of the first king of Israel (over 1,000 years before the present era— 1 Samuel 16:23). King Saul is said to have felt "refreshed" and "well" and free from distress after his music therapy sessions, although this feeling was not long lasting. Music is valuable not only for those who seek relaxation, but is also a useful intervention for those experiencing dementia. It improves their social behavior, speech, and moods exhibited.[511]

Meditation

Many relaxation techniques are available of which meditation is one. The strategy involves focusing on subjects other than the stressful experience. Some meditation strategies can be recommended to the Christian, but others are unhelpful. Those that are not recommended to Christians are commonly based on Eastern philosophies and practice and often involve a mystical experience.[512] Mind-emptying experiences, for which these philosophies are well-known, are inherently dangerous, as the Scriptures are not backward in telling us. The famous story told by Jesus of an individual emptying the mind, but filling it with nothing, stands as a warning. The man's latter state was far worse than his commencing point, as he had ostensibly passed the point of no return to a normal and God-fearing life through his neglect (Matthew 12:43–45). If any might think to dismiss the activity of spirits in our modern world, then personal accounts of missionaries and the testimony of those who have been rescued from slavery to evil spirits should sober anyone.[513]

Christian meditation is thoughtful or active contemplative rather than mind emptying; it is a time when one considers the meaning of God's revelations to humans, particularly through the life and teachings of Jesus Christ. During meditation, time is given to prayer when appeal is made to illumination of the word by the Holy Spirit (John 14:26; 16:13).[514]

Some find it helpful to journal their thoughts after reading, thinking, and praying about a Bible passage.

Rest, Relaxation, and Social Interaction

Children-parent relationships that are warm and nurturing aid in the balanced development of children and reduce stress in their lives and condition the response of these individuals to stress later in life. On a broader basis, a well-known emotional approach to stress management is to provide social interaction and support. This may involve family, friends, and others such as church groups. Studies consistently have shown that social support decreases the release of stress hormones, improves immune response, and reduces morbidity and mortality.[515]

Interest in the possible mechanism for a positive response to befriending and tending behavior has focused on the hormone oxytocin. When positive social contact occurs, the flow of this hormone is increased and this is associated with reduced anxiety and moderated stress responses. Other chemicals may mediate the positive outcome as well, such as opioids.[516]

One proven method of relaxation in a supportive social setting is honoring the rest day that God set aside at creation (Genesis 2:2–3). The seventh-day Sabbath (Saturday) was set aside at creation to allow communication with God (meditation, prayer, and rejoicing) and joining with others in group activities—family and like-minded people (Exodus 20:8–11).[517] Millions find this experience relaxing, rewarding, and stress relieving. They feel comfortable worshiping on this day for the added reason that all the alternatives are institutions created by humans. A genuine spiritual experience has proven health benefits.[518]

> *One proven method of relaxation in a supportive social setting is honoring the rest day that God set aside at creation.*

Life Transformation

Seeking a new direction in life and peace with God and humanity are well tested pathways to find meaning, comfort, and closeness to God. When positive outcomes are realized through these endeavors, stress is reduced and the participant enjoys better health.[519]

The psalmist David tells us something of his search for spiritual renewal after wandering from God (Psalm 32:1–5). The steps involved in achieving spiritual growth are several.[520] The first involves reflection on one's life and considering who we are and why we are here. In the Christian context, this leads us to a realization that we are valuable in God's sight, for the simple but profound reason that Jesus offered His life to purchase our salvation. In considering this amazing sacrifice, we are urged to give unreserved devotion in return. We respond first by repentance and confession (forgiveness follows immediately) so that closeness to the divine is felt. This step is pictured in the Bible as sweeping the rooms of the mind clear, which must be followed by filling it with new insights and sharpening our thoughts about the direction of our lives (Matthew 12:43–45). The believer is obedient to the moral principles of God's kingdom as an outcome of this faith experience. The final piece of the process is sharing the experience of joy and the insights gained with others, bonding in a community of believers (Hebrews 10:24–25), and participating in meaningful group activities (Malachi 3:16).

Exercise

Regular exercise not only has physical but also psychological and emotional benefits when it is enjoyed. Anxiety and depression are reduced and self-image, work accuracy, and speed are improved. A physiological basis has been proposed for the improved sense of well-being. One theory suggests that endorphins are released during short-term exercise events, which give rise to a euphoric state. Whatever the mechanism, it has been shown consistently that those who exercise daily perceive less stress in their lives. They are protected from more dangerous effects of stress.[521]

The human body was designed for activity, and the progenitors of the human race were given regular work assignments to ensure their continued physical, psychological, and emotional health (Genesis 2:15, cf. 3:19).

Highlight: *Some relaxation techniques that can be recommended are humor, music, exercise, and meditation on spiritual themes.*

Guiding Principles and Practical Suggestions

1. Injurious effects are observed on the human body when stress hormone levels are elevated for abnormal periods of time.

2. Uncontrolled stress predisposes to coronary heart disease and gastrointestinal problems. It also influences the immune system and reduces its ability to combat various diseases.

3. Coping skills increase with practice. Active involvement in resolving stress leads to success.

4. Attitude adjustment is significant to resolving stress through accepting responsibility, expanding the field of possible solutions, and being optimistic about the resolution of the situation.

5. Behavior modification can occur when there is a desire to change and conscious choice is made at the point of action to substitute a more appropriate alternative. The Christian is at an advantage in that the person can confidently ask for God's help.

6. Creative problem solving aids in relieving stress. Thinking beyond the usual ways in seeking solutions can be rewarding.

7. Communication skills are significant to forming effective relationships. Effective communication involves both self-disclosure and listening. Conflicts may arise when poor communication occurs. The most effective ways in which conflict can be resolved is through the use of persuasion and dialogue.

8. Putting wrongs right with our colleagues and confessing our fault to God is an excellent way in which to relieve stress.

9. Effective time management calls for prioritizing tasks and scheduling activities. The importance of balancing work and personal time is significant in managing stress.

10. If anger is not controlled, it will harm one's health. Anger can be managed through changing the work environment and also by modifying one's attitude. Forgiveness is a good way to commence the process of coping with the stress of anger.

11. Prayer is a serious coping device. It functions to give hope and fosters optimism and lowers anxiety. It involves talking to God as a friend.

12. Relaxation techniques to lessen stress are humor, music, meditation, hydrotherapy, and other devices.

13. Introducing a spiritual dimension to life and seeking a transformational experience can have a positive impact on stress reduction.

Section III: Spiritual Health

Memorable Quotes[522]

"Belief affects biology"
(Norman Cousins).

"The weak can never forgive.
Forgiveness is the attribute of the strong"
(Mohandas Gandhi).

"They who know the truth are not equal to
those who love it, and they who love it are not
equal to those who delight in it"
(Confucius).

"Forgiveness does not change the past,
but it does enlarge the future"
(Paul Boese).

"Where love is, there God is also"
(Mohandas Gandhi).

"Confidence and hope
do more good than physic"
(Galen).

"Without faith, hope and trust, there is no promise for the future, and without a promising future, life has no direction, no meaning and no justification"
(Adlin Sinclair).

"And now abide faith, hope, love, these three; but the greatest of these is love"
(1 Corinthians 13:13).

"For I know the thoughts that I think toward you, says the Lord, thoughts of peace and not of evil, to give you a future and a hope"
(Jeremiah 29:11).

"For it is by grace you have been saved, through faith—and this not from yourselves, it is the gift of God"
(Ephesians 2:8, NIV).

"I have come that they may have life, and that they may have it more abundantly"
(John 10:10).

"This (Christ) was the true light that gives light to every man who comes into the world"
(John 1:9, NIV—footnote).

Chapter 11

Purpose and Certainty

The optimism that accompanied life just before the present time (the modern era) was supported by advances made through application of the scientific method. The modern era began when individuals attempted to understand the world through observation, experimentation, and reason. From this experience, laws, hypotheses, and values were derived and many new inventions came to our aid. Some regarded the acquisition of such knowledge as heralding a golden era of accomplishment and the alleviation of human misery. As a consequence, a new purpose seized the imagination of many. The era commenced from a largely Christian base and credit was given to God, but at least in recent years, advances are commonly regarded as being wholly derived through human effort. This is not surprising since the scientific method specifically eliminates God from any place in the worldview generated. Today there is a marked contrast between a belief that gives sympathetic attention to the words delivered by God (contained in Bible) and those who argue with its words or the atheist who discounts the idea that the document is special. The impact of these later movements is noticed immediately when it comes to concepts concerning the purpose of life and the value attributed to spirituality.

The optimistic response characteristic of the modern era has been blunted in recent years as human misery, environmental degradation, wars, and other woes have continued. Now we find that many have rejected modernism and with it the appeal to reason and the acceptance of absolute truths. The postmodern individual holds that so-called scientific facts are interpretations of truth and that we can only convey relative truth through language. Postmodern enthusiasts reject the idea of absolute moral principles. They seek to experience personal freedom and pleasure as foremost priorities. Chaos and shallowness may be embraced and the value of human beings may be brought to the level of other living organisms or lower.[523]

In this supposedly brave new world, it is held that the only requirement for peaceful coexistence among humans is mutual tolerance. However, the fragility of this approach is illustrated by the demands made by postmodernists for sensitivity, tolerance, and justice. They forget that all these positions involve clear moral values.[524] Postmodern theorists do not seek to establish a worldview but rather seek to argue that there is no foundation for such viewpoints.[525] Postmodernism actually proclaims a loss of identity and holds the idea that human life is characterized by "plurality and ambiguity." Postmodernism represents a "complex spiritual condition."[526] Indeed, it is the concept of spirituality and what it contributes to health that I wish to explore in this chapter. Many scientists are realizing that spirituality has its own health benefits.

> *Spiritual health is...the next frontier to be understood, appreciated, and practiced so as to improve the health status of peoples around the world.*

Spiritual health is a much discussed topic and is the next frontier to be understood, appreciated, and practiced so as to improve the health status of peoples around the world. It should interest us that the World Health Organization regards spiritual well-being as a component of mental health. The idea is that "one of the most important ways

spirituality contributes to human value is that it tends to define the human being in a way that is beyond merely the ability to function."[527] Some of the ways in which human beings are defined by their spiritual understandings deal with the meaning and purpose of life and a sense of harmony with self and God. Spiritual care contributes to the healing process.[528]

Purpose has a solid connection with the concept of origins. It is noticed that the worldview adopted will give rise to either an optimistic or pessimistic outlook. In the evolutionary model, for example, human life ultimately is destined to end in oblivion unless successful escape to and colonization of another planet is contrived.[529] The outlook for the Christian believer is much more positive. The creator and redeemer, Jesus Christ, is coming again to remake this world and populate the globe with redeemed individuals dedicated to a universal, unchangeable moral code. Such a view brings a tangible spiritual dimension to living and this, medical science indicates, gives rise to superior health outcomes.

The health benefits of a spiritual dimension have intrigued scientific research groups; in fact, the positive contribution to health is very strong.[530] Today, in the world of exchange of ideas, we notice that a number of philosophies give suggestions for improvement to our well-being. For example, the Buddhist position on suffering has something to offer us in that it holds that ignorance is an important contributor to suffering and that knowledge is liberating.[531] Some Christians find abundant support for the position that it is knowledge in the physical, intellectual, social, and spiritual domains that is essential to an understanding of vibrant health.[532] A number of comparative studies have considered the relationship of religious involvement to well-being. Indeed, individuals who experienced religious involvement showed lower mortality. Perhaps not surprisingly, there are differences in response depending on religious orientation with Christians showing more positive relationships than Buddhists or Taoists, for example.[533]

Highlights:

1. *Spiritual health is a significant contributor to human well-being.*

2. *Postmodern thought signals a loss of identity and purpose.*

3. *Purpose in life is connected with concepts about origins. Christian belief gives the clearest view of value and purpose.*

Health Benefits of Spirituality

As indicated already, there is no serious suggestion that spirituality can be ignored when happiness and well-being are considered. Interestingly, the more serious an individual's connection with religion and spirituality, the greater the benefit to well-being observed.[534]

Now, it has been suggested that our health is affected to the degree that our needs are met in regards to the meaning and purpose of life, love and belonging, and hope and forgiveness.[535] I will discuss some of these ideas in this section.

Purpose of Life

The evolutionary model of origins holds, in its purest form, that "the universe we observe had precisely the properties we should expect if there is, at bottom, no design, no purpose, no evil and no good, nothing but pitiless indifference."[536] This means that the human race is here by chance and is destined to a cruel and purposeless existence over the full scope of its uncertain history. The theory asserts that at some time life arose from non-life by random events and then other forms of life came into being as a result of adaptations and natural selection (involving bloodshed, cruelty, and pain) to finally give rise to apes and then humans as an unplanned outcome. In short the theory is an attempt to explain everything by relying on natural phenomena. On account of this, it excludes any need for the presence of a Superior Being in the life-generating process.[537]

It is the sense of meaninglessness for the existence of both the universe and human beings that challenges all religions to investigate the claims of evolution. If we are simply machines to propagate our genetic material in a self-sustaining process[538] or a "chemical scum" in the vast universe or a "trivial, accidental embellishment to the physical world"[539] then we are of all creatures most miserable and are basically a selfish race. Those who champion such ideas have to admit that evil, pain, and suffering are essential to human evolution and will continue to have their place. On account of these ideas, there is perhaps no prospect of a brighter future or indeed of a distant future at all.[540]

The theory goes on to assert that the emerging human line eventually developed social behavior. Clearly, since this line ultimately evolved from simpler, non-social animals, this is the only option available. This step also poses a problem. Darwinian theory considers that individual fitness is of utmost importance for evolutionary success. It further considers that social behavior was highly significant in the development of human intelligence and that social behaviors were developed in the primates.[541] These developments were problematic in that individuals engaging in cooperative acts could perhaps better spend their energies courting females and begetting progeny or in gathering resources. However, the favored idea is that these individuals, by assisting kin-relationships, were indeed helping themselves. After all, any cost to the giver is actually beneficial to the survival of the helper's own genes in the group. In addition, the shared genes of interest are increased in future generations.[542] This means that, for evolutionary theorists, any prosocial behavior observed is driven by survival and kinship considerations, which are basically selfish.

Highlights:

1. *Evolutionary theory declares that life as we see it today can be accounted for by chance and the expression of the principle of the survival of the fittest.*

2. *Existence ultimately is meaningless, and humans are driven by selfish motives like other animals.*

An alternative and well-developed view holds that the human race was created by God in a singular, purposeful act at the end of the creation of the biological world. He made Adam and gave him a companion, Eve; they were made in a noble form. They were given the specific tasks of populating and caring for the earth (Genesis 1:26–28; 2:15, 20). From the beginning humans were social creatures with the capacity to love, and they had all other living creatures under their direction and care (Genesis 1:28; Ps 8:4–9). The human pair was designated to meet restfully together in a social gathering with God on the seventh day, which He specifically made for relaxation and worship. God set the example of acceptable social behavior in the Garden of Eden by meeting together with the human couple on a regular basis (Genesis 2:2, 3; cf. Exodus 20:8–11). Another designated purpose in the existence of humanity was to communicate, learn from, and socialize with God and the angels, and establish a new order of beings on this earth to bring glory to God.

> *The human pair was designated to meet restfully together in a social gathering with God on the seventh day.*

Humans soon faltered and failed to fulfill God's purpose; in other words, antisocial behavior arose. The loss of innocence of the first human pair was on account of their disobedience and lack of trust in their creator. They succumbed to the temptation to disobey God along the lines suggested by Satan, an evil angel. He was expelled from heaven for his rebellious activities there (Genesis 3:1; Revelation 12:7–9). Subsequent to Adam and Eve following Satan's suggestions, they argued among themselves over who was to blame for the unfortunate events that led to their disobedience (Genesis 3:1–13). They both ended up indirectly putting the blame on God. In other words, self was put above God. Now, in order to rescue individuals from the consequences of disobedience—eternal death—Christ, the creator, died for the human race, the just for the unjust (1 Peter 3:18). This loving act pales all others and established the worth of sinful human beings.[543] This account tells us that all are equal by both creation and redemption.

The apostle Peter is clear that those who call themselves Christians will show this conviction in their socially responsible behavior. Dedicated Christians are empathetic or show "compassion" and are "tender-hearted" because they have experienced the love of God. They will return good comments in exchange for evil words. This is a clear break with the first inclinations of many (1 Peter 3:8–9). Antisocial behavior is not in the thinking of Christians for they are law abiders and peacemakers (Matthew 5:9; Romans 13:1–3). The Christian has an elevated view of purpose for the Scripture calls them "ambassadors for Christ" (2 Corinthians 5:20). They also joyfully share with others their experience of freedom from guilt and the love and peace that God gives. They show through their lives and testify to the magnificent qualities of Christ's character.[544] They are interested and active in preserving the works of God in nature, for they understand that nature speaks about God's attributes (Romans 1:20; Revelation 11:18).

Prosocial behavior found in Christians is driven ultimately by a realization that humans share a common origin and all have been offered the gift of eternal life through the loving act of Christ. Hence, such behavior represents a joyful response to the mercy offered and is a statement of dedication to share such understanding with others. In fact, the overriding purpose of such believers is to share the good news about their origins and salvation (literally "vibrant health" derived from the Latin word *salus*) with others (Matthew 28:19, 20; Hebrews 1:1–3).

It should not surprise us after this preamble that scientists have found, among those who identified a spiritual dimension in their lives, a greater sense of meaning and purpose. In fact, 93 percent of studies (45) showed a positive relationship.[545]

Highlights:

1. *Christian belief holds that humans were created through a singular, creative act by a personal God. He made them social beings who were designed to act cooperatively.*

2. *Disobedience to God's will has brought suffering, but Christ's saving grace (love) has given all incredible value.*

Belonging and Love

We all desire to belong. Even the famous vagabonds of Denmark, who specialize in being marginal, non-conformist, unemployed members of society, have an annual vagabond family reunion.[546] At this event, held once a year, they even crown their own king. This gives them pride and a sense of identity among kindred spirits.

Every society has its initiation ceremonies, its own valued rites of passage into the different levels of responsibility as children and young people progress through the various stages of maturity. These rites of passage give and reinforce the feeling of value in the individual and their role in society. The group is thus given solidarity and the initiates have a new and mature view of the world and accept new rights and obligations.[547]

In modern society, we may suffer from a loss of identity and a sense of self-worth. On account of this, some are opting out of life. The diminishing role of religion and the resulting confusion about moral values and behavior has added to the sense of uncertainty.[548]

The need to belong is fundamental with humanity. Fulfillment of this need is required for balanced emotional, social, and ego development.[549] This need to belong has been experienced by humanity over recorded history. To illustrate, there is a story in ancient Hebrew literature of the first murder committed by a man named Cain. As a result of his act, he was isolated from segments of society. He recoiled from the isolation that his own actions had brought and considered that his exclusion from socializing with many of his kinsmen was more than he could bear (Genesis 4:12, 13).

God created humans as social beings, as individuals who would be happy to communicate with their Creator and thus have an overwhelming sense of belonging. He specifically set aside one day of the week (Saturday) to commemorate His commitment to humanity and to give all who wished to respond a new sense of identity (Genesis 2:2, 3; Exodus 31:16, 17; Isaiah 56:1–8; Ezekiel 20:12). Herein lies the special contribution of Christianity, it tells us how we might fellowship with God on the basis of His "freely giving and forgiving love." It is not through any virtuous living that we gain God's approval to fellowship but simply through our need of His love. He loves "because it is His nature to love." This sets Christianity apart from all other religions and accounts for its attractiveness. The believer does not perform acts of goodness or penance to gain merit. The only question of practical value is: "Will we be won by such love?"[550]

Highlight: The need to belong is fundamental with humanity. Christian belief assures us of belonging and of being valued.

The love that God offers, He alone possesses.

The love that God offers, He alone possesses. It was given a special name in the early Greek manuscripts and is known as *agape*. The features of this love are: it does not depend on anything that humanity has done; it is indifferent to value, which means no one is excluded irrespective of their past (Matthew 5:45); it is creative, which means that an individual of no apparent worth is given value by such love (2 Corinthians 5:17–21; Ephesians 4:20–24); and it is the initiator of fellowship with God, for He offers unworthy humanity fellowship, forgiveness, and love (John 3:16).[551]

The existence of God's outrageous love (*agape*), and the reason why it was revealed in a spectacular fashion in the life of Jesus Christ on earth, resolves the question asked by skeptics and philosophers about the presence of evil and suffering. During Christ's life on earth, the originator of evil, Satan, was shown to operate by a defective set of ideas and to lack mercy. It was shown that he is responsible for destruction, suffering, and unhappiness in the world and is incapable of love (Job 1:8–21; 2:2–8; Revelation 20:7–10; 21:4). On the other hand, God's righteous character was fully displayed by Christ's suffering and death (mercy) on behalf of the misdeeds of the human race (Romans 5:5–8; 9:14–16). His character was shown to be wonderful and unique. His kingdom was shown to be based on a code of justice that has eternal application and that is compatible with His display of mercy (Psalm 89:14).

The outcomes of such understandings are several. First, Christians with a clear understanding of God's love wish to communicate this idea to all irrespective of position, race, or religious creed (Matthew 28:19, 20; Revelation 14:6, 7). Sometimes these qualities are shown. For example, in

a study of Christian college students who identified with Christ's teachings at a deep-seated level (intrinsic), they showed tolerance and sociable behavior. However, religious belief is often associated with social distancing behavior and prejudice toward selected groups.[552] Secondly, believers have an excellent basis for hope even when struck by illness, accident, and misfortune. Such hope is free to all those who accept the existence of Christ's provisions of saving mercy and love.

Highlight: *God's outrageous love (**agape**) shown in the sacrifice of Christ for humanity served to illustrate the righteous principles of His government and draws all people to acknowledge the beauty of His character.*

Hope

Human history is scattered with the deeds of men and women who have thought to make a difference because they are fired by the hope of a better future. Some have even sacrificed their lives to this end. The names of several individuals come to mind whom have shown great force of personality and have acted a critical role in stopping some of the worst excesses in human exploitation. William Wilberforce in Britain was a powerful force in the abolition of slavery, and Nelson Mandela was central to the abolition of apartheid in South Africa.

The world has seen many religious and political leaders come and go who have hoped for an ideal world where peace, justice, cooperation, and equality are evident everywhere and where human creativity can be experienced fully. Indeed, in all the experiences of life, we hope and work for a good outcome. Hope is also a vital dimension in recovery from illness, bereavement, and challenging experiences in our lives. It is the construct that carries many buoyantly through life for they look forward with hope to life beyond the grave.

The concept of hope I use here carries with it two prominent and complementary ideas. The first is that the view of the future presented is desirable, and the second is that there is a possibility of the concept being realized.[553]

The first element of hope I wish to develop relates to *desirable outcomes*. There have been many fine examples of people fired by thoughts of achieving desirable outcomes. When Earnest Shackleton's 1914 expedition to the Antarctic ended with his ship being crushed in pack ice, he was challenged to save his men who by now were marooned on inhospitable Elephant Island. With no means of communicating with the outside world but with this hope burning strongly, he set out in a small boat with a handful of companions on a perilous sea journey covering 1,333 kilometers (720 nautical miles) to South Georgia Island. They then were challenged with a treacherous trek overland through unexplored terrain to seek help for colleagues at a whaling station. It then took four successive rescue attempts stretching over 100 days to retrieve the stranded men. They had gone through a terrible ordeal, but they made preparations for their rescue every day, buoyed by the hope that the "Boss" might return today. He came suddenly during favorable weather, and in less than an hour the survivors were plucked to safety. This rescue was fueled by hope on both sides. It created history written in "letters of fire" and turned Shackleton's failure into a glorious example of self-sacrifice and courage.[554]

Hope drives political and military endeavors, and there is perhaps no better current example of the former than President Obama's reflection on desirable outcomes for the United States political landscape. He expressed this sentiment in his pre-election book *The Audacity of Hope* where he spoke of his plans to bring a divided country together. The book strikes a clear note of hope and optimism. High expectations of success give rise to the emotion of lively hope. Hope is a positive emotion that can be nurtured particularly by attention to the spiritual side of human nature.[555]

In the Christian context, desirable outcomes always come to the fore. These are conceived at multiple levels. The first is that an enduring experience with Christ is a sure remedy for guilt and for healing broken human relationships (Psalm 32:1; Proverbs 28:13; Romans 4:7; Philippians 2:3; James 3:13–17). The second area of hopefulness relates to promises of success in helping others escape from eternal oblivion by sharing the gospel with them (Matthew 28:19, 20; 2 Corinthians 5:18–21). The third area of hope relates to the final delivery of believers from the presence of sin and suffering to be with God in a world made new (Romans 8:22–25; Revelation 21:1–4).

Highlight: *Hope-filled individuals seek and work toward achieving desirable outcomes and share the view that there are reasonable expectations for success.*

The second element to the concept of hope (or the prospects of realization of the object of hope) is related to *assurance and faith*, when we speak of it in a Christian context. Remember the text that says: "Now faith is the *assurance* of *things* hoped for, the conviction of things not seen" (Hebrews 11:1, NASB). In Christianity, assurance is found in the person who has divided time (BC/AD/BCE). Christ is accepted as having lived and died. Except for the most hardened skeptic, these facts are acknowledged. Even atheists are among the group of believers on this point.[556] The issue is not Christ's life and death, but His resurrection. The apostles and disciples of Christ did not question His resurrection, as many met and talked with Him. The opposition, reviling, imprisonment, and cruel deaths that many of them suffered on Christ's account motivated them to examine carefully the evidences for their faith. Their careful examination of these facts did not alter their constancy, patience, and courage. They simply found no evidence that the facts about Jesus' life and resurrection were false. The opposers of the Christian church were eager to find evidence but could not offer any credible proof that Jesus did not rise from the dead. If this had been possible, the church would have fallen into disarray. But the church expanded on its persuasive merits and not by means of the sword.[557]

The opposers of the Christian church were eager to find evidence but could not offer any credible proof that Jesus did not rise from the dead.

Assurance

Christians can afford to be assured, for they passionately consider that their God is eternal, a person of impeccable truthfulness, and who is coming again to take His followers to their heavenly home. Their salvation is assured. This belief is based first on the certainty of Christ's life on earth, which is an undisputed historic fact, and on the evidences of His resurrection.[558] The fulfillment of prophecy adds an objective positive note that can be tested against the evidences of history. In addition, the reality of the Christian experience, which is affirmed by believers around the globe and in every age, brings a personal assurance that cannot be contested effectively (2 Peter 1:16–19). Having introduced the idea of prophecy, I will illustrate how powerful this can be in reinforcing assurance and optimism.

There is a challenging prophecy on the succession of significant world empires found in Christian literature that identifies the political and religious forces that would have a determining influence on selected world events from the prophet Daniel's time until the coming of Christ. In the account given

by the prophet, he was shown a great image whose head represented Babylon and the chest and thighs the two succeeding kingdoms. The fourth kingdom of iron was represented by the legs. Finally, the feet were shown as being composed of iron and clay, and these kingdoms will disappear at Christ's coming (Daniel 2). Daniel had been informed and indeed lived to see Babylon succeeded by Medo-Persia (Daniel 5:29–31). From greater detail subsequently given to him, he knew that the third kingdom would be Greece (Daniel 8:20, 21). Every history book affirms the prominent nations that followed Babylon were Medo-Persia and Greece. The fourth empire was the iron monarchy of Rome. This was the empire functioning during Jesus' time on earth (Luke 2:1–7). The western part of the Roman Empire broke up in AD 476.[559] The prophecy predicted that the empire would be completely fragmented. Various national groups emerged, just as the prophecy predicted.[560] Many other prophecies are given, and clear fulfillment can be shown adding to the weight of evidence. All this gives firm confidence in God's Word and His promises, but it does not eliminate the need for faith.

Faith

In the study of spirituality and health, investigators say that hope involves "connectedness with something greater than the self."[561] I have encompassed this dimension in our discussion under the heading of faith. Now the mental transaction that we call faith does not represent a blind endeavor but is built on reason and evidence. Faith is something that is not unique to the religious realm. For example, there are certain scientific beliefs that are not "susceptible to proof," a point made forcibly by Thomas H. Huxley many years ago. In science it must be assumed that the law of causation operates at all times and under all circumstances, which cannot be proven. There are other unprovable assumptions. Science is not a faith-free enterprise. In fact, every worldview has faith elements.[562]

Faith is something that is not unique to the religious realm.

Religious faith is multi-dimensional and, if understood and experienced, brings an individual to a state of quiet confidence (trust) in the spiritual realm and leads to a change in the life and to continuing loyalty (obedience).[563] Christians focus their attention on the person of Jesus Christ. Confidence in Him is not entirely apart from reason (e.g., Isaiah 1:18, 1 Thessalonians 5:21),[564] for it is based on the evidences of history, nature, and human experience. It is relatively easy to believe the historical facts about Jesus; it is more difficult to accept that He is the creator of the universe, on the evidence that we can see or reason about, and somewhat more difficult to move beyond this point. This is where the more intangible element of faith comes into operation (2 Corinthians 5:7). Such an exercise gives meaning to life (something that science is incapable of achieving), and it fills in the missing pieces of the picture. The concept of unity of knowledge takes on a new dimension.

In the domain of Christianity, we speak of having faith when we develop an overwhelming trust in God. Clearly, such an individual has moved somewhat beyond direct evidences. Perhaps we can liken the experience to that of young people developing a relationship that blossoms into commitment in marriage. As these folk get to hear the account of the other person's life and take on information about their character that comes from personal observation and their reactions to other people, they begin to believe that each is genuine and that the qualities they see are admirable. This conclusion is reinforced if their friends and family share their assessments.

At the end of this process, they are willing to commit or trust their lives to each other until death parts them. They cannot see the future clearly, but they trust that the qualities of character they have observed will carry them through both the good times and the bad. These qualities may include such things as kindness, reasonableness, even temper, optimistic approach, and dependability. These qualities and more define the person who acts through the principle of love. Having seen the evidence of such love, we can trust in the future performance of our partner. The same is true in the experience of the Christian.

Faith in Jesus Christ is built upon the idea that he sacrificed His life for the salvation (vibrant health) of the human race in an act of unselfish love. No greater act of sacrifice is possible for humans than to give one's life for another.[565] This act of salvation carries with it the related idea that Christ is coming again to rescue those who trust in Him so that they can live with Him in heaven and subsequently inhabit a new earth free from disease, pain, disaster, and death. Faith also recognizes that believers cannot save themselves, for they are mortal.

Having accepted Jesus' amazing demonstration of love,[566] we then can move forward and accept His further claims. He asserts that He can change our lives in a remarkable fashion. Those who have tested these waters know that their requests are answered when they ask in faith. When they confess their sins, they have peace, for they believe their sins are forgiven. When they pray for strength to overcome temptations, it is given. This trust is carried into everyday life and aids in facing its difficulties. Ask those who have gone down this track, and they will tell you that it is not a delusion but that the experience is real.[567] This is what we call faith, for it moves beyond the evidence. The individual trusts in God's promises and claims them.

There is an important distinction between faith and presumption. The presumptive individual does not offer obedience to God or offers only partial obedience (cf. Matthew 7:21–27). This is in marked contrast to the person of faith who is obedient to all the revealed will of God. The difference between faith and presumption can be illustrated by reference to an interesting story involving the king of Prussia, Frederick the Great. He was intent on creating a thirty-meter high fountain. Frederick asked the mathematician Leonhard Euler to tell him how this spectacle could be achieved, for it had not been accomplished previously. Euler duly considered the problem and delivered his verdict, but the king was determined to take a short cut. Perhaps not surprisingly, the fountain did not live up to its promise, and the king blamed the distinguished mathematician for the failure of the enterprise. Now, more than 250 years later, Euler has been exonerated for giving the correct advice.[568] The king wished to claim the reward for the money he had spent after failing to comply with the conditions laid down by the planner, Euler. In like manner, God's promises are ours to claim when we wholeheartedly follow His will for us. We will speak of the will of God in the next chapter.

Highlight: The Christian has an assurance that God's Word and His promises are true through understanding Bible prophecy and experiencing the changes that acceptance of divine help brings to the conduct of everyday life.

Optimism Benefits Health Outcomes

Anticipation of desirable outcomes and optimism impact physical health. For example, medical researchers have discovered that there is a connection between a person's mood and stress hormone levels. It has been found that looking forward to a humorous video will give rise to a positive mood even before the experience. This state of positive anticipation leads to a decrease in the negative stress hormones and to an increase in beneficial ones and promotes the prevention and/or healing of disease. Norman Cousins, whose experience in

humor therapy led to the emergence of the science of psychoneurobiology (emerging field of immunology), said that curative outcomes "flow out of an individual's capacity to retain an optimistic belief and attitude toward problems and human affairs in general." Furthermore, in his view it is a "perversion of rationalism to argue that words like 'hope' or 'faith' or 'love' or 'grace' [and laughter] are without physiological significance. The benevolent emotions are necessary not just because they are pleasant, but because they are regenerative."[569]

One fascinating outcome of studies involving spirituality is that individuals who have a sense that they are "working cooperatively with God" have a clear advantage over those who do not have such a connection. Believers showed fewer issues with alcohol and nicotine addiction, and substance abusers who experienced religious faith were more optimistic and showed higher resilience to stress. The outstanding benefit for individuals with a spiritual orientation was improved mental and physical health.[570]

Highlight: An optimistic approach to life has observable health benefits.

Guiding Principles and Practical Suggestions

1. Modern thinking, with its appeal to reason, is being replaced by postmodern ideas. In this view, scientific information is considered relative truth because it is conveyed through language. The emphasis of many postmodern individuals is on personal freedom and pleasure; in fact, they display a complex spiritual condition.

2. Spirituality is the next frontier to be conquered. The sense of ultimate meaning and value is vitally connected to health outcomes. Spiritual well-being is regarded by some experts as a vital component of mental health.

Purpose of Life

3. One of the ways in which human beings are defined by their spiritual understanding involves the question of the purpose of life. This inevitably involves the question of origins.

4. The theory of evolution offers the human race an assurance that it is here by chance and is destined to a cruel and purposeless existence over the full scope of its uncertain history.

5. An alternative and well-developed view holds that humanity was created by God in a singular, purposeful act at the end of the creation of the biological world.

6. In the creation view, the newly created humans were given the specific tasks of populating and caring for the earth. Another designated purpose in the existence of humans was to communicate, learn from, and socialize with God, and to establish a new order of beings on this earth to bring glory to God.

7. Subsequent to creation, humans decided to rebel against God. In turn, God provided a way to rescue humanity from eternal death through the sacrifice and ministry of Jesus. Those who accept this salvation have an elevated view of purpose for the Scripture calls them "ambassadors for Christ." They joyfully share with others their experience of freedom from guilt and the love and peace that God gives. They also are interested and active in preserving the works of God in nature, for they understand that nature speaks of Him.

Belonging and Love

8. A sense of belonging and love are connected to spiritual health. God created humans as social beings, as individuals who would be happy to communicate with their creator and thus have an overwhelming sense of belonging. He specifically set aside one day of the week (Saturday) to commemorate His commitment to humanity and to give all who wished to respond a new sense of identity. Now we are invited to fellowship with God on the basis of His "freely giving and forgiving love."

Hope

9. Christian philosophy is pervaded by the concepts of hope, love, grace, and faith. Each individual is given worth by God's love demonstrated through Christ's death. God offers abundant forgiveness and love, and this is the basis of the vibrant hope seen.

10. Christians can afford to be optimistic and assured. Their belief is based first on the certainty of Christ's life on earth, which is an undisputed historic fact, and the reality of the Christian experience, which brings personal assurance.

11. Confidence in God is not entirely apart from reason, for it is based on the evidences of history, nature, and human experience. Reason is not simply the domain of science; it is encouraged in religion as well.

12. Faith is a necessary part of the spiritual experience. It moves beyond the evidence. The individual trusts in God's promises and claims them. Faith, by its very nature, demands that the individual who claims God's promises also undertakes to perform His will.

13. Hope represents a vital dimension in the recovery from illness, bereavement, and challenging experiences in our lives.

14. A state of positive anticipation and optimism leads to a decrease in negative stress hormones and to an increase in beneficial ones and promotes the prevention and/or healing of disease.

Chapter 12

Being Good Neighbors

Nobel Peace Prize recipients have been nominated in most years since 1901, indicating that we live in a world where being a good neighbor is constantly needed and valued. Inequalities, ethnic and religious tensions, and the unilateral furthering of national and sectional aspirations are often at the heart of international neighborhood disputes.

Some of the achievements of peacemakers have been remarkable, such as Desmund Tutu's role in the peaceful resolution of the apartheid issue in South Africa. Commenting on his achievement, Egil Aarvik, chairman of the Norwegian Nobel Committee, stated of the man who never learned to hate:

Desmond Tutu has shown that to campaign for the cause of peace is not a question of silent acceptance, but rather of arousing consciences and a sense of indignation, strengthening the will and inspiring the human spirit so that it recognizes both its own value and its power of victory. To this fight for peace we give our affirmative 'yes' today.

Racial discrimination can never be anything but an expression of shameful contempt for humankind. Racial discrimination used and defended as a political system is totally incompatible with human civilization. This year's Peace Prize is therefore an attempt to awaken consciences. It is, and has to be, an illusion that privileged groups can maintain their position through repression.

That such things can have a place in our future is a lie which nobody should allow themselves to believe…. We feel ourselves united with him (Tutu) in the belief in the creative power of love. With his warm hearted Christian faith he is a representative of the best in us all. [571]

Our ability to live in harmony is linked to our worldview and the value we place on human life. Many views exist and some lead to better understandings of the value and dignity of human beings than others. I will look at two extremes in order to illustrate my statement.

Worldview Does Matter

The dominant view of origins held in the Western world, and which is widely accepted elsewhere, is the evolutionary theory. This worldview is expounded upon by New Atheists in their attempt to explain how life arose on earth without recourse to the notion of a creator being involved. Some of its most insistent advocates tell us frankly that "evolution is a selfish doctrine." This is on account of the individual seeking their own welfare in order to "gain a selective edge" in accordance with the idea that tooth, claw, and the shedding of blood are the prerequisites for evolutionary success. "Selfishness is taken to characterize the life at the deepest level" for we are simply "robot vehicles blindly programmed to preserve selfish molecules known as genes."[572]

Evolution is a selfish doctrine.

In the social context, the operation of the doctrine of survival of the fittest is expressed in the cut and thrust among human beings observed in the marketplace. In order to bolster acceptance of the theory, it is not surprising that sociobiologists have focused on the competition

seen in the natural world rather than on examples of cooperation. This bias is in accordance with the demands of evolutionary theory. And it should not astound us that they are unable to recognize genuine examples of altruism.[573] The end result of such intellectual activity is that the individual is regarded as a machine and has "no meaning, no purpose, no significance." It follows that the question of right or wrong is not particularly relevant. Self-interest dominates the thinking of believers of such a worldview. However, among all this there is a wistful longing for less selfish outcomes.[574]

The self-interest that consumes many who wish to understand that life arose by chance will be contrasted here with the view held by selected Christian (those which take the Bible literally) and Islamic groups. They believe that life is a gift from the hand of a personal, infinite creator God and that humankind was created deliberately and not through the process of evolution. The special Christian view is that at the outset people had value because he was created in God's moral image. However, he did not honor the trust placed in him by the creator and rebelled, hence defacing humanity's most valuable asset. Now, humanity's abnormal act of rebelling against God releases His maker from blame as the originator of evil in this world. This means that morals have a solid basis, for God is shown to be good and not the author of evil. Indeed, "God's character is the moral absolute of the universe." Moreover, the beauty of His character is still evident in the substitutionary death of Christ for the guilt of the human race.[575]

Highlight: Worldview influences behavior. The evolutionary view is based on the operation of selfish motives. The special creation view is based on the concept of love.

In the next section I will deal with the uniqueness and value of humans and then discuss some moral guidelines widely recognized among national groups.

Uniqueness and Value of Humans

The unique characteristic of humans resides in the enormous intellectual capacity possessed and the associated language ability and ethical behavior.[576] Not all are willing to agree that this capacity was a design feature but rather insist that it is a matter of random evolutionary events over vast periods of time. If humans do not have a unique place among living organisms, then it can be argued that there is nothing particularly sacred about human life and that animals are entitled to equal consideration. This is the position taken by Peter Singer and others so that it becomes possible to advocate abortion on demand, infanticide, euthanasia, and other activities.[577]

The gospel confirms the value of humanity and the race's total indebtedness to Christ.

Among Christians alone are those who believe in a God who is personal, infinite, loving, holy, and just. Their God is the creator of the universe and of the human race that was made in His image. On account of this, all humans are unique and have dignity. A short period after creation, the race deliberately rebelled against God, hence defacing the moral image originally given. Jesus Christ intervened in giving His life to rescue sinful individuals from certain destruction. This sacrifice on behalf of the race shows the immense value He places in each individual. The gospel confirms the value of humanity and the race's total indebtedness to Christ. God's giving was an expression of the totally extravagant love known as *agape* or God's love. It represents the ultimate example of goodness.[578]

The Christian God is living (Christ rose from the grave) and offers salvation as a gift to all who will accept it.[579] This means that all humans have equal value. Jesus' disciples are committed to follow His example by treating all with equality.[580] The apologist Anders Nygren explains that *agape* originates with God and believers can act only as channels to show God's love to others. The gift given freely to humanity is cheerfully and willingly passed on to others by believers without distinction.[581]

In the next section, I will discuss the implications of Jesus' gift. It delivers humans from confusion and futile attempts to find moral and ethical values that will function to preserve a just society.

Highlight: Believers understand that a person is unique, has dignity, and has value above all other creatures.

The Law of Nature

Societies value fairness, equality, and the application of principles they feel are right; these values are upheld by law. Values that regulate societal behavior may be rooted in religious beliefs or otherwise depending on the national identity.

The recognition of a "higher ideal of justice" than the laws of state comes from ancient times. In more modern times a famous appeal was made to Natural Law or the law of nature by the World Court at the Nuremburg War Trials, which ultimately resulted in the adoption of the Universal Declaration of Human Rights by the United Nations in 1948.[582]

The idea of there being "a higher law" that transcends national boundaries and that impacts the consciences of men and women has been recognized for millennia (Romans 2:14, 15). Irrespective of the philosophical orientation adopted, there are widely held elements of ethical conduct based on concepts of moral law.[583]

The universality of such understandings has been outlined in some detail by C. S. Lewis.[584] This record shows that there is a striking similarity between the last six principles in the Christian Decalogue and moral behavior widely accepted from ancient to modern times across many cultures. This has led to the suggestion that humans, created in the image of God, respond to laws written in their beings through the operation of reason (Romans 2:14, 15).[585] The standard present at the creation of humanity was formalized subsequently in the Decalogue that was famously given to the prophet Moses on Mount Sinai as a universal code of conduct (Exodus 19:14–20:17).[586] The first four elements of the Decalogue are similarly not without witness. They speak to the invisible qualities of God and are revealed in nature (Psalm 19:1–11; Romans 1:18–22). Ultimately, humans must respond to the call of conscience and to the evidences found in nature for which reason seeks an answer. Now the condemnation of actions meted out by our consciences along the lines of appeals to universal moral principles speaks to the existence of a coming judgment, for law does not stand apart from a judge.[587]

Highlight: The existence of a higher moral law is recognized across cultures and speaks to the existence and character of its originator, God.

Basis of a Moral Life

It has been said that humility and selflessness are the bases of a moral life.[588] Pride and selfishness, the very opposites, are promoted by philosophies that exclude God from their worldview. Indeed, evolutionary theorists, for example, have made nature "a surrogate God" to account for the gaps in the theory.[589] The concept that life arose by random events and then developed progressively through the survival of the fittest or the most well-adapted (which is simply another way of saying

the cruelest and meanest survive) means that the idea of a person relating to others (morals) lacks a definitive anchor point because human heritage by this model is anchored in cruelty. It is not surprising, then, that in the modern way of thinking there is no right or wrong; rather society determines what it is comfortable in tolerating.[590]

Humility and selflessness are the bases of a moral life.

We found in the last section, however, that humans have for millennia entertained ideas that there is right and wrong and, in fact, have developed a reasonable pattern of correspondence across cultures. In the age in which we live, society tends to shun the idea of absolutes of right and wrong, yet continues to deplore the descent of our civilizations into the cruelest behavior. The answer to this dilemma is surely in acknowledging that humans were made in the image of God, had a precise knowledge of the good, and initially delighted in following wholesome ways. However, at a definite point in history, humankind rebelled against the goodness of God and chose evil, and as a consequence became cruel and antisocial. In this pattern of understanding, God is seen as the author of goodness and, in fact, His "character is the moral absolute of the universe" (cf. Genesis 3:1–7; 4:5–15).[591]

This brings us back to consider humility and selflessness as the basis of moral life. The linkage point between humility and selflessness is explained by one writer thus: "love is the agent which He (God) uses to expel sin from the heart. By it He changes pride into humility, and enmity and unbelief into love and faith."[592] It is the love of God that is the basis for moral absolutes because it reflects His character. This is why the Christian scriptures describe God as love (1 John 4:9). Now, this is no ordinary love as pointed out previously.

The Christian religion is different from all others in that God does the giving; Christ died on the cross for sinful, hostile humanity. God did not wait or depend on human achievements, sacrifice, or the gaining of merit; the initiative was with Him. Humanity could not offer anything of value to God. When God's gift is accepted by faith, the human being becomes an agent through whom this special love is shown to others. Such love can only flow to others as the individual gives unlimited devotion to God, for this love depends for its transmission on a vibrant personal relationship being established with the divine (Matthew 5:16).[593]

The concept of God's love (*agape*) gives humankind an anchor point. It answers the questions: Where did I come from? Who am I? What is my destiny? How should I act? God's character is seen as the moral absolute of the universe; He is the author of good and the keeper of it. He has transmitted an account of His goodness to humanity in the life and teachings of Christ (Immanuel—God with us). Christ identified the Decalogue, the Ten Principles delivered by God to Moses at Mount Sinai, as the source of practical information on how to relate to others (Exodus 20:2–17; Matthew 22:36–40). This is not to infer that mere doing is the substance of an acceptable response to God; an appropriate response to God is the acceptance of His gift of love by faith, acknowledging specific shortcomings, asking for God's forgiveness for our unwholesome acts, and depending on Him daily for strength to do good.[594]

Highlights:

1. *The firmest basis for a moral life is to recognize that God is the author of goodness and love and has offered to save rebellious humanity.*

2. *Unselfish love (*agape*) has made salvation possible. It originates with God, gives value to all, and functions as a moral absolute.*

Understanding God's love and its relationship to His character prepares us to act as good neighbors.

Acting as a Good Neighbor

With the recognition that there are absolute moral standards and a personal, infinite creator God who has shown such care for rebellious humanity, a response is required. An appreciation of God's amazing act of dying on behalf of humanity can be shown by responding to such love personally in obedience to God's will and sharing such understandings with others through demonstrating what God's love is like. How this works is illustrated by the famous story told by Christ regarding the Good Samaritan.

This story was related in response to the question from a lawyer about the conditions of inheriting eternal life. Jesus asked the questioner how he understood the matter, and the lawyer answered: "You shall love the Lord your God with all your heart, with all your soul, with all your strength, and with all your mind, and your neighbor as yourself" (Luke 10:27). On the assurance from Jesus that our duty to God cannot be separated from our duty to others (i.e., the first four commandments of the Decalogue are significant and linked to the last six), the lawyer sought to clarify whom his neighbor was. It was then that Jesus told the story of the Good Samaritan. On a journey from Jerusalem to Jericho a traveler was assaulted, robbed, and left injured by the roadside. Two religious leaders came past the man, but they offered no assistance. Then a Samaritan, a member of a race despised by the Jews, came near the victim. Without considering his own safety, the political correctness of the act he was about to do, or what it might cost, he assisted the stranger to a place of help and provided for his care. In answer to the question "Who is my neighbor?" the answer was provided by the story. Our neighbor is anyone in need of our help and bears no relationship to race, religion, or educational standards (Luke 10:30–37).

Christians understand that "practical self-sacrifice for the good of others" is the one criterion that determines whether their name answers to their profession.

Alert Christians understand that "practical self-sacrifice for the good of others" is the one criterion that determines whether their name answers to their profession. The act may simply be a word of cheer or some other deed of mercy, kindness, or love to persons in the family or community. Such behavior comes in response to the love of God that they have experienced.[595] Unselfish love is the most important quality that is shown in a Christian, for without it all the good deeds done and even martyrdom are pointless. Such love indicates that there is a complete devotion to and fellowship with God. Unselfish love is not self-serving and it does not cease to be expressed after a brief, flashy display. It does not give way to impatience and cannot coexist with envy, jealousy, and anger. This love seeks justice and is happy when truth is promoted. Individuals who possess unselfish love are optimistic and trust others (1 Corinthians 13:1–8). They function to make the communities in which they live peaceful and delightful places to live.

Thoughts and acts of kindness are not restricted to those who claim to know God. Those who show kindness in response to the laws of nature and cherish this revelation will receive an honorable, eternal reward from God (Romans 2:12–16).[596] For the more privileged, guidelines have been given whereby such love can be cultivated.

Highlight: Acting as a good neighbor means helping those in need without discrimination. Kind acts, when motivated by a response to Christ's love shown to the believer, establish a firm basis for continual, harmonious relationships in the community.

Cultivation of Christian Love

By reading and understanding the words that God has left us in the Bible we can begin to appreciate the character of God (John 6:53–56, 63). Jesus made this idea exceedingly clear when He stated, "Man shall not live by bread alone, but by every word that proceeds from the mouth of God" (Matthew 4:4). The apostle Paul added to this thought when he stated that all Scripture represents God's inspired word (2 Timothy 3:16).

What we take into the mind will affect our character.

What we take into the mind will affect our character. If we understand this relationship, we will wish to avoid filling the mind with obscene, crude, and trivial things. Instead, we will seek to maintain a close relationship with God by studying His revealed will and the authentic record of His life. The apostle Paul likens the experience to a sharp sword driving into the body (Hebrews 4:12). The good news is, if we do not resist the molding influence of God, our manner of thinking and acting will be changed.

An experience with God that leads to change comes as a result of regular encounters. It is through reading and considering the Word of God that we are changed (Proverbs 2:3–5). Quick encounters, especially where we are not prepared in our minds to accept ideas other than those we wish to find, will not be life changing. Jesus instructed His followers to come with the attitude of learners, asking for God's help so that they might understand His will for them (John 14:26). We should not develop the opposite mistaken idea that the quantity of study we do is important. Rather, it is the consistency and quality of the study, meditation on the word, and the subsequent changes in the life that occur as a result that counts.[597]

Understanding God's Word is intimately connected with prayer. The advice given in the New Testament scriptures is to pray without ceasing (1 Thessalonians 5:17). This does not mean that we become useless on account of praying all the time, but it does indicate a willingness to seek advice from God's book of instructions in our everyday activities and to ask for help in times of special need. What this means is illustrated in the experience of the cupbearer Nehemiah (Nehemiah 2:4). One day while in the Persian court he was looking sad, and the king suspected a plot against his life. In this tense situation, Nehemiah sent a prayer to God as he stood before the king. Wisdom was given to him, and a happy outcome occurred that furthered the interests of his exiled nation.

Prayer is best done in private in order to get away from the distractions of everyday life and to create a special atmosphere; it is not for show. Prayer is the time to speak to God as a friend; hence we do not need to indulge in vain repetitions (Matthew 6:6–15). It is a time when we present specific requests to God, such as asking forgiveness for the sins that have come to our notice (Matthew 6:12; Philippians 4:6). This also is the time to reflect on the direction of our life, on the things that frustrate, and on the areas where improvement might be made. It is a time to reflect on the joys and blessings that God has given.[598]

When we see what God has undertaken and suffered for the salvation of the human race, we want to take advantage of His offer of rescue. The Bible pictures God as a loving father who rejoices when someone comes to knowledge of the gift

He has offered and takes advantage of it. In effect, God has created a loving environment for us so that we can understand the consequences of our sinful actions. He gives us the spirit of repentance (Acts 5:31). As we understand the hideous consequences of disobedience both for this world and other worlds and when we understand God's moral standards, we want to do only those things that please Him. This experience of understanding God's righteousness and plan for our lives will lead us to confess our failings and then ask for guidance and help in our everyday living. God immediately exchanges our guilt with a sense of peace and joy (Romans 5:1, 2).

In the environment we have just mentioned, the conditions are right for our conscience to be educated and to develop. Knowledge and understanding of God's moral code causes us to develop uneasiness about some of our practices.[599] Our internal control mechanism now tells us, "I am ashamed of considering such an action" or "I do not wish to follow this suggestion, as it is not the way Jesus would do it." Taking on specific moral guidelines as our own is called internal attribution—this means that we feel uncomfortable, guilty, or shameful about certain actions, but our motivation to follow the guidelines is not from fear.[600] The Bible talks about this process as "doing the will of God from the heart" (Ephesians 6:6). God wishes us to do things because we find pleasure in obeying His will.

God actually promises to transform our thinking so that we wish to do His will and then He provides us the power to accomplish this (Ezekiel 11:19, 20; Ephesians 3:20, 21). The important thing for us to understand is that the changes that occur in the Christian are accomplished through the merits of Christ and not by the individual (1 Corinthians 1:30, 31; 2 Corinthians 5:21; Hebrews 10:14). A positive attitude is taken by the Christian to the great issues in everyday life. The assurance is that ample provision will be given in all situations. God has given an undertaking that He wishes us to triumph with Christ (Ephesians 6:12–18).

God has given an undertaking that He wishes us to triumph with Christ

---

The response of the Christian to the gift and experience of love will motivate the individual to share this good news with others. The Bible speaks about being ambassadors for God (Matthew 28:19, 20; 2 Corinthians 5:20). Many have responded to this challenge and have done amazing exploits for God. The Bible account of the work of the apostles, particularly Paul, is an outstanding illustration of what this has meant to some. He went on extensive missionary journeys. He, with Barnabas, took the gospel to Syria and Asia Minor. Thus, they commenced the first foreign missionary program and laid the foundation for the survival of the church through the dark ages to come.[601] The apostle Paul was willing to suffer in order to share the good news with others. He counted the experience a privilege. His experience challenges us.

Highlights:

1. *Cultivating Christian love is accomplished through understanding Christ's life, ways, and will and praying for guidance.*

2. *Understanding God's ways leads to repentance and to daily requests for help.*

3. *God promises to change our thinking and to give us a new appreciation for how we might*

serve others and pass on the gift of love we have received from Him.

Guiding Principles and Practical Suggestions

1. Our ability to live together in harmony is linked to our worldview and to the value we place on human life.

2. The evolutionary worldview is widely accepted. It represents a selfish doctrine in which the fittest and meanest survive and in which there is "no meaning, no purpose, no significance." Self-interest dominates such a viewpoint, not compassion or an interest in the welfare of others. Life is considered a game of chance.

3. An alternative worldview is that life is a gift from the hand of a personal, infinite creator God. Humans were deliberately created in the image of God and not through the process of evolution.

4. Humans did not honor the trust placed in them by the Creator, but early rebelled. Nevertheless, their value has been placed beyond question by the sacrifice of Jesus on their behalf.

5. God's giving to rescue humanity can be explained by a totally extravagant love known as *agape* or God's love, which has no equal in the world.

6. God gave humans value by His sacrifice for them and delivered them from confusion and futile attempts to find moral and ethical values. These values have been given to the human race in the Decalogue and function to preserve a just society.

7. Humans were made in the image of God and had a precise knowledge of honorable principles and initially delighted in following these

ways. This explains why universal moral principles (natural law) have been identified. They speak also to the existence of a coming judgment.

8. It is the love of God that is the basis for moral absolutes, for it reflects His character. This is none other than the unconditional love shown by God for lost human beings who do not deserve it. When this gift is accepted by faith, the human being becomes an agent through whom God's love is channelled to others.

9. God has transmitted an account of His goodness to humanity in the life and teachings of Christ (Immanuel—God with us).

10. An appropriate response to God is to accept His gift of love by faith, to ask for His forgiveness for our unwholesome acts, and to depend on Him daily to do good.

11. An appreciation of God's love can be shown by responding in obedience to God's will and sharing such understandings with others through demonstrating what God's love is like.

12. Unselfish love is the most important quality that is shown in a Christian, for without it all the good deeds done and even martyrdom are pointless.

13. Reading and understanding the words that God has left in the Bible lead to an appreciation of the character of God. The reading of God's word must be intimately connected with prayer if it is to be understood.

14. The molding influence of God will be felt in the life if it is not resisted. The way of thinking and doing will be changed as a result.

15. Focused attention to the life and works of Jesus each day leads to spectacular changes. God promises to transform an individual's thinking so that he or she will wish to do His bidding. God provides the power to accomplish the desirable changes.

16. God desires people to accomplish wholesome things because they find pleasure in obeying His will.

17. The Christian joyfully responds to the gift and experience of love by sharing the good news with others like efficient ambassadors. They are happy and experience vibrant mental health as a result.

Endnotes

Introduction

Chapter 1

1   R. Preece, *Sins of the Flesh* (Vancouver: University of British Colombia Press, 2008), 71–91; C. Spencer, *The Heretic's Feast* (London: Fourth Estate, 1993), 38–51, 83, 84.

2   B. W. Ball, *The English Connection* (Cambridge: James Clarke & Co., 1981), 170, 171.

3   Ibid., 5, 84, 160–162, 173.

4   J. Moskala, *Journal of the Adventist Theological Society* 22, no. 2 (2011): 21, 22.

5   Ibid., 12–14, 18, 21.

6   O. Chambers, *My Utmost for His Highest* (Grand Rapids, MI: Discovery House Publishers, 1992), September 1 thought.

7   Ball, *English Connection*, 174, 175.

8   Preece, *Sins of the Flesh*, 35, 36; Spencer, *The Heretic's Feast*, 22.

9   S. Colledge and J. Conolly, eds., *The Origin and Spread of Domestic Plants in Southeast Asia and Europe* (Walnut Creek, CA: Left Coast Press, Inc., 2007), 21–36; A. Sanchez-Mazas et al., eds., *Past Human Migrations in East Asia: Matching Archaeology, Linguistics and Genetics* (New York: Routledge, 2008), 40–83.

10   Spencer, *The Heretic's Feast*, 90.

11   Ibid., 182.

12   Ibid., 118–120.

13   Ibid., 127.

14   A. Roberts and J. Donaldson, eds., *The Ante-Nicene Fathers. Latin Christianity: Its Founder Tertullian* (New York: Charles Scribner's Sons, 1918), Apology 9, 3: 24–26.

15   L. M. Flood, *British Medical Journal* 340 (2010): c164; Spencer, *The Heretic's Feast*, 125, 126.

16   Spencer, *The Heretic's Feast*, 163–172.

Section I: Physical Health

17   Brainy Quotes, http://1ref.us/8k; Thinkexist, http://1ref.us/8l; Quote Garden, http://1ref.us/8n (accessed on June 2, 2015).

Chapter 2

18   F. S. Sizer and E. N. Whitney, *Nutrition: Concepts and Controversies*, 8th ed. (Belmont, CA: Wadsworth/Thomson Learning, 2000), 98–103.

19   T. C. Campbell and T. M. Campbell, *The China Study* (Dallas, TX: Benbella Books, 2006), 95–97; W. J. Craig, *Nutrition and Wellness: A Vegetarian Way to Better Health* (Berrien Springs, MI: Golden Harvest Books, 1999), 27–30; S. J. Simpson and D. Raubenheimer, *Aging* 1, no. 10 (2009): 875–880; Sizer and Whitney, *Nutrition*, 182–187, 197–199; S. M. Solon-Biet et al., *Cell Metabolism* 19 (2014): 418–430.

20   Craig, *Nutrition and Wellness*, 30–39, 267.

21   Ibid., 33–42; L. A. Smolin and M. B. Grosvenor, *Nutrition: Science and Applications*, 4th ed. (New Jersey: John Wiley & Sons, Inc., 2003), 141, 142.

22   Sizer and Whitney, *Nutrition*, 210–251.

23   Ibid., 264–268.

24   Craig, *Nutrition and Wellness*, 9–15; M. Mancini et al., eds., *Nutritional and Metabolic Bases of Cardiovascular Disease* (Chichester, West Sussex: John Wiley & Sons, 2011), 121–123; M. J. Orlich et al., *Journal of the American Association of Internal Medicine* 173, no. 13 (2013): 1–8.

25   M. Chopra et al., *Bulletin of the World Health Organization* 80, no. 12 (2002): 952–958.

26   K. A. Marsh et al., *Medical Journal of Australia* open access 1, suppl. 2 (2012): 7–10; J. Nathan et al., *European Journal of Clinical Nutrition* 51 (1997): 20–25.

27   American Dietetic Association, *Journal of the American Dietetic Association* 109, no. 7 (2009): 1266–1282; D. E. Larson-Meyer, *Vegetarian Sports Nutrition* (Campaign, IL: Human Kinetics, 2007), 10.

28   H. W. Hoogenkamp, *Soy Protein and Formulated Meat Products* (Wallingford, Oxfordshire: CABI Publishing, 2005), 3.

29   American Dietetic Association, *Journal of the American Dietetic Association* (2009); Marsh et al., *Medical Journal of Australia* (2012).

30   Craig, *Nutrition and Wellness*, 27–30, 143, 144, 173.

31   Z. Bano and S. Rajarathnam, *Critical Reviews of Food Science Nutrition* 27, no. 2 (1988): 87–158.

32   S. A. Miller and J. T. Dwyer, *Food Technology* 55 (2001): 42–47; M. G. Wiebe, *Mycologist* 18, no. 1 (2004): 17.

33   Marsh et al., *Medical Journal of Australia* (2012).

34   H. F. Bayes et al., *International Journal of Clinical Practice* 61, no. 5 (2007): 737–747.

35   A. V. Saunders et al., *Medical Journal of Australia* open access 1, suppl. 2 (2012): 22–26.

36   Craig, *Nutrition and Wellness*, 173, 174, 180.

37   American Dietetic Association, *Journal of the American Dietetic Association* (2009).

38   Craig, *Nutrition and Wellness*, 195–199; A. V. Saunders et al., *Medical Journal of Australia* open access, 1, suppl. 2 (2012): 11–16.

39   Craig, *Nutrition and Wellness*, 184–194.

40   A. V. Saunders et al., *Medical Journal of Australia* open access 1, suppl. 2 (2012): 17–21.

41   American Dietetic Association, *Journal of the American Dietetic Association* (2009); J. H. Beattie and I-S. Kwun, *British Journal of Nutrition*, 91 (2004): 177–181; World Health Organization, *Diet, Nutrition and the Prevention of Chronic Disease*, Technical Report Series 916 (Geneva: World Health Organization, 2003), 8.

42   B. D. Hokin and T. Butler, *American Journal of Clinical Nutrition* 70, suppl. 3 (1999): 576S–578S; A. L. Rauma et al., *Journal of Nutrition* 125, no. 10 (1995): 2511–2515; S. P. Stabler and R. H. Allen, *Annual Review of Nutrition* 24 (2004): 299–326.

43   American Dietetic Association, *Journal of the American Dietetic Association* (2009); Craig, *Nutrition and Wellness*, 218; P. C. Dagnelie, *Journal of Nutrition* 127, no. 2 (1997): 379; R. Pawlak et al., *American Lifestyle Medicine* 7 (2013): 60–65; F. Watanabe et al., *Nutrients* 6, no. 5 (2014): 1861–1873; C. L. Zeuschner et al., *Medical Journal of Australia* open access 1, suppl. 2 (2012): 27–32.

44   American Dietetic Association, *Journal of the American Dietetic Association* (2009); Craig, *Nutrition and Wellness*, 215, 218; Pawlak et al., *American Lifestyle Medicine* (2013); Sizer and Whitney, *Nutrition*, 206, 229, 230; The Vegan Society, "B_{12}—Your Key Facts," http://1ref.us/8o (accessed April 27, 2015),.

45   J. F. B. Arendt and E. Nexo, *Clinical Chemistry and Laboratory Medicine* 51, no. 3 (2013): 489–496; G. Mouton, *Nutrition Practitioner*, winter (2008): 1–6.

46   Sizer and Whitney, *Nutrition*, 213–216; E. S. Tee, *Food and Nutrition Bulletin* 23 (2002): 345–348.

47   Sizer and Whitney, *Nutrition*, 227–229; Smolin and Grosvenor, *Nutrition*, 233, 234, 255, 256.

48   P. Sarnsamak, "Health Plan to Make Thai Children Healthier and More Intelligent," *The Nation*, January 8, 2009, http://1ref.us/8p (accessed February 10, 2015).

49   Craig, *Nutrition and Wellness*, 20, 21.

50   American Dietetic Association, *Journal of the American Dietetic Association*

(2009); Craig, *Nutrition and Wellness*, 94–100; R. Edwards, *New Scientist* 181, no. 2430 (2004): 8.

51 Mancini et al., *Cardiovascular Disease*, 79; N. J. Temple et al., eds., *Nutritional Health*, 2nd ed. (Totowa, NJ: Humana Press, 2006), 133–140.

52 United States Department of Agriculture, Center for Nutrition Policy and Promotion, "Dietary guidelines for Americans," 2013, http://1ref.us/8q (accessed February 10, 2015); E. Zacharias, *The Mediterranean Diet: A Clinician's Guide for Patient Care* (New York: Springer Science+Business Media, LLC, 2012), 118, 119.

53 Craig, *Nutrition and Wellness*, 21, 43–46; Mancini et al., *Cardiovascular Disease*, 79; R. E. C. Wildman, ed., *Handbook of Nutraceuticals and Functional Foods*, 2nd ed. (Boca Raton, FL: CRC Press, 2007), 136–138.

54 Craig, *Nutrition and Wellness*, 172, 173; Mancini et al., *Cardiovascular Disease*, 79; F. H. Sakar and Y. Li, *Cancer Investigation* 21 (2003): 817, 818; Sizer and Whitney, *Nutrition*, 424–430.

55 Y-Z. Fang et al., *Nutrition* 18, no. 10 (2002): 872–879; J. T. Kumpulainen and J. T. Salonen, eds., *Natural Antioxidants and Food Quality in Atherosclerosis and Cancer Prevention* (Cambridge: Royal Society of Chemistry, 1996), 36; Mancini et al., *Cardiovascular Disease*, 80; Temple et al., *Nutritional Health*, 173–188.

56 Larson-Meyer, *Vegetarian Sports Nutrition*, 10.

57 R. V. Trauxe, *Emerging Infectious Diseases* 3, no. 4 (1997): 425–434.

58 Craig, *Nutrition and Wellness*, 171–173, 180, 255–258; C. A. Nowson et al., *Medical Journal of Australia* 196, no. 11 (2012): 686, 687; Sizer and Whitney, *Nutrition*, 487–492.

59 Craig, *Nutrition and Wellness*, 255–258.

60 J. L. Hill, *The Case for Vegetarianism: Philosophy for a Small Planet* (Lanham, MD: Rowman & Littlefield, 1996); S. Plamintr, *The Discovery of Buddhism* (Nonthaburi: Write & Read Publishing Co., Ltd, 2007), 146.

61 S. I. McMillen and D. E. Stern, *None of These Diseases*, revised edition (Grand Rapids, MI: Fleming H. Revell, 2000).

62 J. C. Avise, *The Genetic Gods* (Cambridge, MA: Harvard University Press, 1998), 215.

63 Campbell and Campbell, *China Study*, 75–103; World Health Organization, *Chronic Disease* (2003).

64 P. Ellwood et al., *Thorax* 68, no. 4 (2013): 351–360.

65 S. Bacchiocchi, *Wine in the Bible* (Berrien Springs, MI: Biblical Perspectives, 1989), 107–109.

66 Craig, *Nutrition and Wellness*, 103, 104, 172.

67 Ibid., 18.

68 Sizer and Whitney, *Nutrition*, 203.

69 V. Kumar et al., *Robbins Basic Pathology*, 8th ed. (Philadelphia: Saunders, 2007), 314–316.

70 Brainy Quote, http://1ref.us/8r (accessed February 10, 2015).

71 A. Greenhill et al., *Papua New Guinea Medical Symposium*, Goroka, 5–9 September, 2005, 68–69; Food and

Agriculture Organization, "What are mycotoxins?",http://1ref.us/8t (accessed February 10, 2015).

72 A. Atiyyah, "Eat Well, Work Well, Live Well!" http://1ref.us/8u (accessed February 10, 2015); A. Fernando and L. Swidler, *Buddhism Made Plain*, revised edition (New York: Orbis Books, 1990), 27.

73 S. J. Nielsen and B. M. Popkin, *Journal of the American Medical Association* 289, no. 4 (2003): 450–453.

74 P. J. Datta, "India May Soon Overtake China to Become World Diabetes Capital," *The Hindu Business Line*, May 26, 2014, http://1ref.us/8v (accessed February 10, 2015); R. Kannan, "WHO Puts China Ahead of India in Incidence of Diabetes," *The Hindu*, March 22, 2006, http://1ref.us/8w (accessed October 2, 2015); E. S. Tee, *Asia Pacific Journal of Clinical Nutrition* 11, suppl. 8 (2002), S694–S701; T. A. Wadden et al., *Journal of Consulting and Clinical Psychology* 70, no. 3 (2002): 510–525.

75 J. E. Blundell and A. Gillett, *Obesity Research* suppl. 4 (2001): 263S–270S; Nielsen and Popkin, *Journal of the American Medical Association* (2003).

76 D. Martindale, *New Scientist* 177, no. 2380 (2003): 27–29.

77 M. T. Madigan et al., *Brock Biology of Microorganisms*, 10th ed. (Upper Saddle River, NJ: Pearson Education International, 2003), 731–733.

78 Craig, *Nutrition and Wellness*, 150, 151.

79 Campbell and Campbell, *China Study*, 54–60, 95–97.

80 E. C. Knight et al., *Annals of Internal Medicine* 138, no. 6 (2003): 450–467.

81 P. Cohen, *New Scientist* 183, no. 2454 (2004): 15.

82 National Human Genome Research Institute, "Specific Genetic Disorders," 2011, http://1ref.us/8x (accessed February 10, 2015).

83 C. R. Parrish, *Nutrition Issues in Gastroenterology* series 27 (2005): 76–94.

84 S. D. Rampertab and G. E. Mullin, eds., *Celiac Disease* (New York: Springer Science+Business Media, 2014), 123–136.

85 V. T. DeVita et al., eds., *Cancer: Principles & Practice of Oncology* (Philadelphia: Lippincott Williams & Wilkins, 2011), 180, 181.

86 Campbell and Campbell, *China Study*, 73, 74; Solon-Biet et al., *Cell Metabolism* (2014).

Chapter 3

87 G. O'Neill, *Australian Biotechnology News* 2, no. 7 (2003): 18.

88 Craig, *Nutrition and Wellness*, 8, 9.

89 Ibid., 8–15; G. E. Fraser and D. J. Shavlik, *Archives of Internal Medicine* 16, no. 13 (2001): 1645–1652; M. J. Orlich et al., *Journal of the American Medical Association Internal Medicine* 173, no. 13 (2013): 1230–1328; D. Ornish et al., *Lancet Oncology* 14, no. 1 (2013): 1112–1120.

90 W. Turner, "Pythagoras and Pythagoreanism," in *The Catholic Encyclopedia* (New York: Robert Appleton Company, 1911), http://1ref.us/8y (accessed April 25, 2015).

91   K. S. Walters and L. Portness, eds., *Ethical Vegetarianism from Pythagoras to Peter Singer* (New York: Suny Press, 1999), 11–46.

92   C. Chen, *Getting Saved in America* (Princeton, NJ: Princeton University Press, 2008), 78; H. Wu, "Buddhism, health, and healing in a Chinese community," http://1ref.us/8z (accessed February 10, 2015).

93   Mancini et al., *Cardiovascular Disease*, 77, 78; Sizer and Whitney, *Nutrition*, 60, 61.

94   Sizer and Whitney, *Nutrition*, 204; R. A. Stanton, *Medical Journal of Australia* open, 1, suppl. 2 (2012): 5, 6.

95   Craig, *Nutrition and Wellness*, 18–26, 60; Sizer and Whitney, *Nutrition*, 137, 138, 204, 412, 424–430.

96   Medical information is available in the public domain: http://1ref.us/90; http://1ref.us/91; http://1ref.us/92; http://1ref.us/93.

97   Mancini et al., *Cardiovascular Disease*, 81.

98   G. A. Bray, *Journal of Nutrition* 132, no. 11S (2002): 3451S; G. A. Bray, *Primary Care* 30, no. 2 (2003): 281–299; Kumar et al., *Robbins Basic Pathology*, 317.

99   American Association for Cancer Research, "2 Components of Red Meat Combined with Alteration in DNA Repair Increase Risk for Bladder Cancer," http://1ref.us/94 (accessed February 10, 2015); S. A. Bingham et al., *Journal of Nutrition* 132, no. 11 (2002): 3522S–3525S; A. Turbic et al., *Food Additives and Contaminants A* 19, no. 2 (2002): 144–152.

100   Mancini et al., *Cardiovascular Disease*, 81; T. Norat et al., "The Associations between Food, Nutrition and Physical Activity and the Risk of Colorectal Cancer," WCRF/AICR Systematic Literature Review Continuous Update Project Report, October 2010, 102, 103, 124–126, http://1ref.us/95 (accessed February 10, 2015).

101   J. F. Gonzales et al., *Journal of the American College of Nutrition* 33, no. 3 (2014): 239–246.

102   T. E. Moon and M. S. Micozzi, eds., *Nutrition and Cancer Prevention: Investigating the Role of Micronutrients* (Boca Raton, FL: CRC Press, 1989), 13–32; K. A. van der Heijden, ed., *International Food Safety Handbook: Science, International Regulation and Control* (Boca Raton, FL: CRC Press, 1999), 225–238.

103   E. G. White, *The Acts of the Apostles* (Mountain View, CA: Pacific Press Publishing Association, 1911), 191.

104   New South Wales Jewish Board of Deputies, "Kosher Food," http://1ref.us/96 (accessed February 10, 2015).

105   R. A. Laurie, *Meat Science* (Oxford: Pergamon Press, 1968), 123.

106   Campbell and Campbell, *China Study*, 157–182; Gonzales et al., *Journal of the American College of Nutrition* (2014); J. S. Ren et al., *Cancer Epidemiology Biomarkers & Prevention* 21 (2012): 905–915.

107   American Dietetic Association, *Journal of the American Dietetic Association* (2009); Mancini et al., *Cardiovascular Disease*, 81; S. Shankar and R. K. Srivastava, eds., *Nutrition, Diet and*

Cancer (New York: Springer, 2012), 50–52, 295–316; Norat et al., WCRF/AICR Systematic Literature Review, 262.

108 D. P. Burkitt and H. C. Trowell, eds., *Refined Carbohydrate Foods and Disease* (London: Academic Press, 1975), 78, 79, 113–131, 333–345; Campbell and Campbell, *China Study*, 171–174.

109 American Dietetic Association, *Journal of the American Dietetic Association* (2009).

110 American Diabetes Association, http://1ref.us/97 (accessed April 26, 2015); American Diabetes Association, *Diabetes Care* 25, suppl. 1 (2002): S64; Craig, *Nutrition and Wellness*, 147–149; G. L. Khor, *Asia Pacific Journal of Clinical Nutrition* 13, suppl. (2004): S22; Mancini et al., *Cardiovascular Disease*, 133–136; S. Mathur et al., *Diabetes as a Cause of Death, Australia, 1997 and 1998* (Canberra: Australian Institute of Health and Welfare, 2000), ix–xi, 1; M. D. Niculescu and P. Haggarty, eds., *Nutrition in Epigenetics* (Chichester, West Sussex: Blackwell Publishing, Ltd, 2011), 276.

111 N. A. Campbell et al., *Essential Biology with Physiology* (San Francisco: Benjamin Cummings, 2004), 553, 554; Craig, *Nutrition and Wellness*, 146; L. Portetsky, ed., *Principles of Diabetes Mellitus* (Boston: Kluwer Academic Publications, 2002), 39–42.

112 R. Hillson, *Diabetes: A New Guide* (London: Positive Health Guide, 1993), 56–67.

113 American Dietetic Association, *Journal of the American Dietetic Association* (2009); J. Gear et al., *British Medical Journal* 281 (1980): 1415; D. Snowdon and R. Phillips, *American Journal of Public Health* 75 (1985): 507.

114 J. T. Daugirdas, ed., *Handbook of Chronic Kidney Disease Management* (Philadelphia: Wolters Kluwer/Lippincott Williams & Wilkins Health, 2011), 152–158; J. D. Lane, *Journal of Caffeine Research* 1, no. 1 (2011): 23–28.

115 GI Website, http://1ref.us/98 (accessed April 26, 2015).

116 Craig, *Nutrition and Wellness*, 151; J. M. Hannan et al., *British Journal of Nutrition* 97, no. 3 (2007): 514–521; Mancini et al., *Cardiovascular Disease*, 110; B. McCleary and L. Prosky, eds., *Advanced Dietary Fibre Technology* (London: Blackwell Science Ltd., 2001), 162–167.

117 Mancini et al., *Cardiovascular Disease*, 77, 78; R. B. Singh et al., *Cardiology Research and Practice* (2010): doi:10;4061/2010/824938.

118 C. S. Dayrit, *Philippine Journal of Cardiology* 31, no. 3 (2003): 97–104; F. B. Hu et al., *Journal of the American College of Nutrition* 20, no. 1 (2001): 5–19; Mancini et al., *Cardiovascular Disease*, 77, 78; P. W. Siri-Tarino et al., *American Journal of Clinical Nutrition* 91, no. 3 (2010): 535–546.

119 T. H. Applewhite, ed., *Proceedings of the World Conference on Lauric Oils: Sources, Processing, and Applications* (Boulder, CO: AOCS Press, 1994), 99.

120 L. Eyres et al., *Food New Zealand* 14, no. 6 (2014): 17–19.

121 S. Mukherjee and A. Mitra, *Journal of Human Ecology* 26, no. 3 (2009): 197–203.

122   T. K. Xian et al., *Evidence-Based Complementary and Alternative Medicine* (2012): doi:11551/2012/828170.

123   J. M. Arbonés-Mainar et al., *Atherosclerosis* 194, no. 2 (2007): 372–382.

124   Craig, *Nutrition and Wellness*, 60–64, 76, 77, 96, 97; D. J. Pehowich et al., *West Indian Medical Journal* 49 (2000): 128–133.

125   R. R. S. Packard and P. Libby, *Clinical Chemistry* 54, no. 1 (2008): 24–38.

126   R. A. Koeth et al., *Nature Medicine* 19 (2013): 576–585; Mancini et al., *Cardiovascular Disease*, 78, 79.

127   Daugirdas, *Chronic Kidney Disease*, 152–156.

128   Craig, *Nutrition and Wellness*, 85.

129   C. Alarcorn de la Lastra et al., *Current Pharmaceutical Design* 7, no. 10 (2001): 933–950.

130   Craig, *Nutrition and Wellness*, 62–77; Smolin and Grosvenor, *Nutrition*, 343–345.

131   Mancini et al., *Cardiovascular Disease*, 124–128.

132   Ellwood, *Thorax* (2013).

133   V. E. Archer and D. W. Jones, *Medical Hypotheses* 59, no. 2 (2002): 450–457; R. P. Dikshit et al., *Indian Journal of Medical and Paediatric Oncology* 32, no. 1 (2011): 3–11; L. Li et al., *Modern Preventive Medicine*, 36, no. 17 (2009): 3209–3211; I. Serra et al., *International Journal of Cancer* 102, no. 4 (2002): 407–411.

134   M. R. Adams and M. O. Moss, *Food Microbiology* (Cambridge: Royal Society of Chemistry, 1997), 145; A. D. Hocking et al., eds., *Foodborne Microorganisms of Public Health Significance*, 5th ed. (North Sydney: Australian Institute of Food Science and Technology Inc., 1997), 187, 241, 318, 344, 345, 610; R. V. Tauxe, *Emerging Infectious Diseases* 3 (1997): 427.

135   A. Rahman et al., *Journal of Pathogens* (2011): 1–11, doi:10.4061/2011/239391.

136   M. D. Ford et al., *Clinical Toxicology* (Philadelphia: W. B. Saunders Company, 2001), 964–968; B. W. Halsted, *Poisonous and Venomous Marine Animals of the World* (Washington, DC: United States Printing Office, 1967), 2, 21, 27, 699; C. K. Woo and S. L. Bahna, *Clinical and Translational Allergy* 1, no. 3 (2011): 7.

137   H. Shuvel, *Journal of Water and Health* 1, no. 2 (2003): 53–64.

138   R. Shamsi, "Why Islam Forbids Pork?" Yahoo Answers, http://1ref.us/9c (accessed April 26, 2015).

139   J. M. Goldsmid, *Australian Microbiology* 2, no. 5 (1982): 5.

140   E. Young, *New Scientist* 187, no. 2508 (2005): 17.

141   C. J. Barnard and J. M. Behnke, eds., *Parasitism and Host Behaviour* (London: Taylor & Francis Ltd, 2005), 273–281; F. Bruschi, *Journal of Infection in Developing Countries* 6, no. 3 (2012): 216–222.

142   F. Bruschi and K. D. Murrell, *Postgraduate Medical Journal* 78 (2002): 15–22.

143   Barnard and Behnke, *Parasitism and Host Behaviour*, 273–281.

144   J. Flegr et al., *BMC Infectious Diseases* 9 (2009): 72; L. Gilbert, *Microbiology Australia*, 29, no. 4

(2008): 188–190; S. A. Henriquez et al., *Neuroimmunomodulation* 16 (2009): 122–133; J. Randerson, *New Scientist* 176, no. 2366 (2002): 41–43; E. F. Torrey and R. H. Yolken, *Emerging Infectious Diseases* 9, no. 11 (2003): 1375–1380.

145   American Cancer Society, "Recombinant Bovine Growth Hormone," http://1ref. us/9d (accessed February 10, 2015); American Public Health Association, "Opposition to the Use of Hormone Growth Promoters in Beef and Dairy Cattle Production," http://1ref.us/9e (accessed February 10, 2015); G. L. Solomon, *Environmental Health Perspective* 102, no. 98 (1994): 632–635.

146   European Commission, "Hormones in Meat," http://1ref.us/9f (accessed February 19, 2015); R. Johnson and C. E. Hanrahan, "The U.S.-EU Beef Hormone Dispute. Congressional Research Service," http://1ref.us/9g (accessed February 10, 2015).

147   A. Barrett, "The Controversy over Added Hormones in Meat and Dairy," http://1ref.us/9h (accessed February 10, 2015); Solomon, *Environmental Health Perspective* (1994).

148   J. R. Gillespie, *Modern Livestock & Poultry Production*, 7th ed. (Stamford, CT: Cengage Learning, 2004), 137, 138.

149   S. J. Forsythe, *The Microbiology of Safe Food* (Oxford: Blackwell Science, 2000), 70–72; A. Gupta et al., *Emerging Infectious Diseases* 10 (2004): 1102–1109; P. F. McDermott et al., *Journal of Infectious Diseases* 185 (2002): 837–840.

150   P. Hughes and J. Heritage, "Antibiotic Growth-Promoters in Food Animals," http://1ref.us/9i (accessed February 10, 2015).

151   K. Hoffmann-Sommergruber and K. Dorsch-Häsler, *Medical Issues Related to Genetically Modified Plants of Relevance to Switzerland* (Zürich: vdf Hochschulverlag AG, ETH, 2012), 15–19, 22, 26–28; M. Pillay et al., eds., *Genetics, Genomics and Breeding of Bananas* (Boca Raton, FL: CRC Press, 2012), 281–297; World Health Organization, *Chronic Disease* (2003): 8.

152   S. O. Duke et al., *Journal of Agricultural and Food Chemistry* 60 (2012): 10375–10397; G-E. Séralini et al., *Environmental Sciences Europe* 26 (2014): 14, doi:10.1186/s12302-014-0014-5.

153   A. Coghlan, *New Scientist* 175, no. 2354 (2002): 4, 5; P. Cohen, *New Scientist* 176, no. 2370 (2002): 7; Hoffmann-Sommergruber and Dorsch-Häsler, *Medical Issues*; B-R Lu, *Collection of Biosafety Reviews* 4 (2008): 66–141; Smolin and Grosvenor, *Nutrition*, 255, 256, 510; A. Spök et al., *Trends in Biotechnology* 26, no. 9 (2008): 506–517.

154   A. K. Lilley et al., *Trends in Biotechnology* 24, no. 1 (2006): 9–14.

155   Hoffmann-Sommergruber and Dorsch-Häsler, *Medical Issues*, 20, 21; Temple et al., *Nutritional Health*, 373–386.

156   S-W. Choi and S. Friso, *Advances in Nutrition* 1 (2010): 8–16.

157   Ibid., 14; M. D. Niculescu, *ILAR Journal* 53, no. 3/4 (2012): 270–278.

158   C. M. Hassler et al., *Current Atherosclerosis Reports* 2, no. 6 (2000): 467–475; C. S. Patch et al., *Vascular Health Risk Management* 2, no. 2 (2006): 157–162.

159   Bacchiocchi, *Wine in the Bible*, 243–246.

160   K. P. L. Bhat and J. M. Pezzuto, *New York Academy of Sciences* 957 (2002): 210–229; Craig, *Nutrition and Wellness*, 90, 120.

161   N. Labinskyy et al., *Current Medicinal Chemistry* 13, no. 9 (2006): 989–996; M. P. Mattson and A. Cheng, *Trends in Neurosciences* 29 (2006): 632–639.

162   Mancini et al., *Cardiovascular Disease*, 423–426.

163   R. Corder et al., *Nature* 444 (2006): 566.

164   G. Rimbach et al., *Genes and Nutrition* 6, no. 1 (2011): 1–3.

165   American Heart Association, "Alcoholic and Cardiovascular Disease," http://1ref.us/9j (accessed February 10, 2015).

166   National Cancer Institute, "Alcohol and Cancer Risk," http://1ref.us/ax (accessed June 7, 2015).

167   Zacharias, *Mediterranean Diet*, 153.

168   M. V. Holmes et al., *British Medical Journal* (2014): 349, http://1ref.us/9l; C. S. Knott et al., *British Medical Journal* (2015): 350, http://1ref.us/9m.

169   American Dietetic Association, *Journal of the American Dietetic Association* (2009); Y. Z. Fang et al., *Nutrition* 18, no. 10 (2002): 872–879; B. Halliwell and J. M. C. Gutteridge, *Free Radicals in Biology and Medicine*, 3rd ed. (Oxford: Oxford University Press, 1999), 761–767; Mattson and Cheng, *Trends in Neurosciences* (2006).

170   Campbell and Campbell, *China Study*, 102, 103.

171   Gonzales et al., *Journal of the American College of Nutrition* (2014); K. Shetty, ed., *Food Biotechnology*, 2nd ed. (Boca Raton, FL: CRC Press, 2006), 771–778.

172   Niculescu & Haggarty, *Nutrition in Epigenetics*, 252.

173   Craig, *Nutrition and Wellness*, 84; A. V. Rao, *Experimental Biology and Medicine* 227, no. 10 (2002): 908–913; E. Giovannucci, *Journal of the National Cancer Institute* 91, no. 4 (1999): 317–331; Mancini et al., *Cardiovascular Disease*, 172, 173; P. R. Trumbo, *Journal of Nutrition* 135, no. 8 (2005): 20605–20615.

174   E. Giovannucci, *Journal of the National Cancer Institute* 91, no. 4 (1999): 317–331; S. M. Talbott and K. Hughes, *The Health Professional's Guide to Dietary Supplements* (Philadelphia: Lippincott, Williams & Wilkins, 2007), 297.

175   S. A. Hulea, *An Introduction to Vitamins, Minerals and Oxidative Stress* (Boca Raton, FL: Universal Publishers, 2008), 197; C. Remacle and B. Reusens, eds., *Functional Foods, Ageing and Degenerative Disease* (Boca Raton, FL: CRC Press LLC, 2004), 17–22.

176   K. Ge and G. Yang, *American Journal of Clinical Nutrition* 57, suppl. 2 (1993): 259S–263S; A. Melse-Boonstra et al., *American Journal of Clinical Nutrition* 68 (1998): 636–641; World Health Organization, *Chronic Disease* (2003), 8.

177   P. C. Calder and S. Kew, *British Journal of Nutrition* 88, suppl. 2 (2002): S165–S177; Kumpulainen and Salonen, *Natural Antioxidants*, 110; M. Serafini, *International Journal of Developmental Neuroscience* 18, issues 4–5 (2000): 401–410.

178 Craig, *Nutrition and Wellness*, 202–206, 213–219.

179 S. P. Stabler and R. H. Allen, *Annual Review of Nutrition* 24 (2004): 299–326; F. Watanabe, *Experimental Biology and Medicine* 232, no. 10 (2007): 1266–1274; Zeuschner et al., *Medical Journal of Australia* open access (2012).

180 W. Siems et al., *The FASEB Journal* 16, no. 10 (2002): 1289–1291.

181 V. Krishna, *Texbook of Pathology* (Chennai: Orient Longman Private Limited, 2004), 407.

182 D. J. Hanson, "History of alcohol and drinking around the world," http://1ref.us/9n (accessed February 10, 2015).

183 M. S. Bonkowski et al., *Proceedings of the National Academy of Sciences USA* 103 (2006): 7901–7905.

184 M. W. Rajala and P. E. Scherer, *Endocrinology* 144 (2003): 3765–3773.

185 A. P. Gomes et al., *Cell* 155 (2013): 1624–1638.

186 C. Rice, *Becoming Women: The Embodied Self in Image Culture* (Toronto: University of Toronto Press, 2014), 171–175.

187 S. A. Rathus and S. Longmuir, *HDEV*, Canadian edition (Toronto: Nelson Education Ltd, 2012), 211, 212.

188 J. W. Rosenthal and W. J. Carey, eds., *Prevention of Cancer: New Research* (New York: Nova Science Publishers, Inc., 2008), 40, 41; J. Russo, ed., *Environment and Breast Cancer* (New York: Springer Science+Business Media, LLC, 2011), 30–37.

189 World Cancer Research Fund, "Red and Processed Meat and Cancer Prevention," http://1ref.us/9o (accessed February 10, 2015).

Chapter 4

190 C. Levinthal, *Drugs, Behavior, and Modern Society* (Boston: Allyn and Bacon, 1996), 205, 206.

191 A. Betts, *Archaeological Diggings* December02/January 03 (2003); 13–15; C. P. Bryan, trans., *The Papyrus Ebers* (London: Geoffrey Bles, 1930), 162; Levinthal, *Drugs*, 101, 102, 107.

192 Betts, *Archaeological Diggings*, 15; commonly available Sudafed PE contains phenylephrine. Sudafed may be a prescription drug—Dr. N. Walters, personal communications.

193 F. Barron et al., *Scientific American* 210, no. 4 (1964): 29–37; R. P. T. Davenport-Hines, *The Pursuit of Oblivion: a Global History of Narcotics* (London: Weidenfeld & Nicolson, 2001).

194 Levinthal, *Drugs*, 314–316, 324–327.

195 D. K. Arora, ed., *Handbook of Fungal Biotechnology*, 2nd revised ed. (Boca Raton, FL: CRC Press, 2004), 221; P. Kalač and P. Krausová, *Food Chemistry* 90, issues 1–2 (2004): 219–230; H. M. Wallace, *Biochemical Society Transactions* 35, part 2 (2007): 293, 294.

196 R. Fine, *The Meaning of Love* (Hoboken, NJ: John Wiley & Sons, Inc., 1985), 49.

197 J. A. Corsica and M. L. Pelchat, *Current Opinion in Gastroenterology* 26, no. 2 (2010): 165–169; J. Fortuna, *Journal of Psychoactive Drugs* 42, no. 2 (2010): 147–151; P. M. Miller, ed., *Principles of Addiction* (Waltham, MA: Academic Press, 2013), 1: 788–793.

198   M. D. Lemonick, *Time*, Australia, January 20, no. 2 (2003), 43.

199   G. F. Koob and M. Le Moal, *Science* 278 (1997): 52–58.

200   P. W. Kalivas and N. D. Volkow, *American Psychiatric Association* 162 (2007): 1403–1413; E. J. Nestler, *Trends in Pharmaceutical Sciences* 25, no. 4 (2004): 210–218.

201   Levinthal, *Drugs*, 212–216, 295–300.

202   Islamic Research Foundation International, Inc., "Smoking in Islam," http://1ref.us/9p (accessed April 27, 2015); A. A. Sulaiman, *Research on Humanities and Social Sciences* 3, no. 4 (2013): 76–81.

203   Kumar et al., *Robbins Basic Pathology*, 290.

204   National Health and Medical Research Council, *Australian Guidelines to Reduce Health Risks from Drinking Alcohol* (Canberra: National Health and Medical Research Council, 2009); M. H. Winstanley et al., *Medical Journal of Australia* 194, no. 9 (2011): 479–482; World Health Organization, "Alcohol drinking," *International Agency for Research on Cancer* 44 (1998), http://1ref.us/9q (accessed April 26, 2015).

205   P. J. Brooks and S. Zakhari, *Alcoholism: Clinical and Experimental Research* 37, no. 1 (2013): 23–30.

206   M. Bernstein and A. Schmidt Luggen, *Nutrition for the Older Adult* (Burlington, MA: Jones & Bartlett Publishers, Inc., 2011), 271–273; D. M. Hayes et al., *Alcoholism: Clinical and Experimental Research* 37, no. 3 (2013): 425–434; T. Hillemacher, *Alcohol and Alcoholism* 46,

no. 3 (2011): 224–230; S. D. Shukla et al., *Alcoholism: Clinical and Experimental Research* 37, no. 4 (2013): 550–557.

207   M. D. De Bellis et al., *American Journal of Psychiatry* 158, no. 5 (2001): 820–821; S. Maier and J. R. West, *Alcohol Research & Health* 25, no. 3 (2001): 168–174; J. A. Obernier et al., *Pharmacology, Biochemistry, and Behavior* 72, no. 3 (2002): 521–532; S. F. Tapert and S. A. Brown, *Journal of the International Neuropsychology Society* 5, no. 6 (1999): 481–493.

208   N. S. Bryan, ed., *Food, Nutrition and the Nitric Oxide Pathway* (Lancaster, PA: DEStech Publications, Inc., 2010), 118, 119; Mancini et al., *Cardiovascular Disease*, 368–374, 321–326.

209   Mancini et al., *Cardiovascular Disease*, 332–334.

210   Ibid., 427–433.

211   L. H. Opie and S. Lecour, *European Heart Journal* 28, no. 14 (2007): 1683–1693; S. Renaud et al., *Lancet* 339, no. 8808 (1992): 1523–1526.

212   J. Burns et al., *Journal of Agricultural and Food Chemistry* 50 (2002): 3337–3340.

213   J. Ferrières, *Heart* 90, no. 1 (2004): 107–111.

214   M. de Lorgeril et al., *Lancet* 343, no. 8911 (1994): 1454–1459; R. B. Singh et al., *Lancet* 360, no. 9344 (2002): 1455–1461.

215   P. Rozin et al., *Appetite* 33 (1999): 163–180.

216   A. M. White and H. S. Swartzwelder, *Recent Developments in Alcoholism* 17 (2005): 161–176.

217   Inter-Islam, 1998–2001, "The Harms

of Alcohol," http://1ref.us/ay (accessed February 10, 2015).

218 Seventh-day Adventist Church Statements, "Historic Stand for Temperance Principles and Acceptance of Donations Statement Impacts Social Change" (2010): 114, 115, http://1ref.us/9r (accessed February 10, 2015).

219 F. P. Rice, *The Adolescent: Development, Relationships, and Culture*, 9th ed. (Boston: Allyn and Bacon, 1999), 439, 440; J. White and R. Humeniuk, *Alcohol Misuse and Violence: Exploring the Relationship* (Canberra: Australian Government Publishing Service, 1994), 4, 5, 10, 11.

220 J. F. Ashton and R. S. Laura, *Uncorked! The Hidden Hazards of Alcohol* (Warburton, Victoria: Signs Publishing Company, 2004); Kumar et al., *Robbins Basic Pathology*, 290, 291.

221 Hanson, "History of alcohol and drinking around the world."

222 Bacchiocchi, *Wine in the Bible*, 54–74, 106–128.

223 M. Ryan, *Sports Nutrition for Endurance*, 2nd ed. (Boulder, CO: Velo Press, 2007), 9.

224 A. Marshall, *The R.S.V. Interlinear Greek-English New Testament* (London: Samuel Bagster and Sons Limited, 1978), 755; J. S. Morton, *Science in the Bible* (Chicago: Moody Press, 1978), 89–91; R. Young, *Analytical Concordance to the Holy Bible* (London: Lutterworth Press, 1975), 916 on the Greek words *pharmakeia* and *pharmakos* translated as sorcerer.

225 Chen, *Getting Saved*, 78; D. Uloom, "Islam and Drugs," http://1ref.us/9s (accessed February 10, 2015).

226 Kumar et al., *Robbins Basic Pathology*, 295, 296.

227 R. B. Kanarek and H. R. Lieberman, eds., *Diet, Brain, Behavior: Practical Considerations* (Boca Raton, FL: CRC Press, 2012), 7.

228 American Water Works Association, *Waterborne Pathogens* (Denver, CO: American Water Works Association, 2006); P. Ravenscroft et al., *Arsenic Pollution: A Global Synthesis* (Chichester, West Sussex: Wiley-Blackwell, 2009).

229 Craig, *Nutrition and Wellness*, 343–350.

230 J. Chan et al., *American Journal of Epidemiology* 155, no. 9 (2002): 827–833; Ryan, *Sports Nutrition*, 7.

231 J. Ciabattoni, *Doctor C's Medical Guide: What You Need to Know* (Bloomington, IN: Xlibris Corporation, 2009), 270; A. Hindle and A. Coates, eds., *Nursing Care of Older People* (Oxford: Oxford University Press, 2011), 169; M. Nair and I. Peate, eds., *Fundamentals of Applied Pathophysiology* (Chichester, West Sussex: John Wiley & Sons, 2009), 451; M. Secher and P. Ritz, *Journal of Nutrition, Health and Aging* 16, no. 4 (2012): 325–329.

232 Kumar et al., *Robbins Basic Pathology*, 7, 13.

233 H. P. Rang et al., *Pharmacology*, 5th ed. (Philadelphia: Churchill Livingstone, 2003), 599–601.

234 T. N. Kelly et al., *Stroke* 39 (2008): 1688.

235 C. H. Ashton, *British Journal of Psychiatry* 178 (2001): 101–106; Kumar et al., *Robbins Basic Pathology*, 297.

236 E. Cardeña and M. Winkelman, eds., *Altered Consciousness: Multidisciplinary*

Perspectives (Santa Barbara, CA: Praeger, 2011), 1: 30–31; Kanarek & Lieberman, *Diet, Brain, Behavior,* 273,274; B. B. Fredholm et al., *Pharmacological Reviews* 51, no. 1 (1999): 83–133.

237   J. V. Higdon and B. Frei, *Critical Reviews in Food Science and Nutrition* 46, no. 2 (2006): 101–123.

238   B. D. Smith et al., *Caffeine and Activation Theory: Effects on Health and Behavior* (Boca Raton, FL: CRC Press, 2007), 284–294.

239   I. C. W. Arts and P. C. H. Hollman, *American Journal of Clinical Nutrition* 81, no. 1 (2005): 3175–3255; E. J. Topol, ed., *Textbook of Cardiovascular Medicine,* 3rd ed. (Philadelphia: Lippincott Williams & Wilkins, 2007), 93–132.

240   J. M. Hodgson and K. D. Croft, *Molecular Aspects of Medicine* 31, no. 6 (2010): 495–502.

241   S. Egert and G. Rimbach, *Advances in Nutrition* 2 (2011): 8–14.

242   L. Chan et al., *Food Research International* 51, no. 2 (2013): 564–570; J. E. Hallanger Johnson et al., *Mayo Clinic Proceedings* 82, no. 6 (2007): 719–724.

243   A. L. Kristjansson et al., *Journal of Caffeine Research* 1, no. 1 (2011): 75–82.

244   K. A. Clauson et al., *Journal of the American Pharmacists Association* 48, no. 3 (2008): E55–63; N. Gunja and J. A. Brown, *Medical Journal of Australia* 196, no. 1 (2012): 46–49; M. O'Brien et al., *Academic Emergency Medicine* 15, no. 5 (2008): 453–460.

245   K. E. Miller, *Journal of Adolescent Health* 43, no. 5 (2008): 490–497; K. E. Miller and B. M. Quigley, *Journal of*

Caffeine Research 1, no. 1 (2011): 67–73; C. J. Reissig et al., *Drug and Alcohol Dependence* 99, no. 1–3 (2008): 1–10.

246   B. M. Cohen and W. A. Carlezon, *American Journal of Psychiatry* 164 (2007): 543–546.

247   Hanson, "History of alcohol and drinking around the world."

248   Rice, *The Adolescent,* 252–255; M. Szalavitz, *New Scientist* 176, no. 2370 (2002): 40.

249   Y. Al-Qaradawi, "Islam Probibits Alcohol and Drugs," http://1ref.us/9t (accessed February 10, 2015); Plamintr, *Discovery of Buddhism,* 148–152.

250   R. J. Shephard, *Aerobic Fitness & Health* (Champaign, IL: Kinetics Publishers, 1994), 220, 232–268; E. Singer, *New Scientist* 180, no. 2421 (2003): 8.

251   Temple et al., *Nutritional Health,* 34–47.

252   Craig, *Nutrition and Wellness,* 7–15, 213–219.

253   J. Joseph et al., *Journal of Neuroscience* 29, no. 14 (2009): 12795–12801.

254   D. R. Shaffer, *Social & Personality Development,* 3rd ed. (Pacific Grove, CA: Brooks/Cole Publishing Company, 1994), 227–233, 430–432.

255   C. A. Anderson et al., *Psychological Bulletin* 136, no. 2 (2010): 151–173; H. Phillips, *New Scientist* 194, no. 2600 (2007): 33–37; Rice, *The Adolescent,* 252–255, 309–311; J. P. Rushton, *Altruism, Socialization, and Society* (Englewood Cliffs, NJ: Prentice-Hall, Inc., 1980), 133–145; T. F. M. ter Bogt et al., *Pediatrics* 131, no. 2 (2013): e380–e389, doi:10.1542/peds.2012-0708.

256   Rushton, *Altruism,* 170–174.

257   B. L. Seaward, *Managing Stress: Principles and Strategies for Health and Wellbeing*, 2nd ed. (London: Jones and Bartlett Publishers, 1997), 309, 310.

258   Seaward, *Managing Stress*, 310, 311, 314, 315; M. Cobb et al., eds., *Oxford Textbook of Spirituality and Healthcare* (Oxford: Oxford University Press, 2012), 362.

259   E. G. White, *The Desire of Ages* (Mountain View, CA: Pacific Press Publishing Association, 1940), 83, 259, 260.

260   Seaward, *Managing Stress*, 310–312, 319.

261   Ibid., 318, 319.

262   M. E. P. Seligman, *Learned Optimism* (Milsons Point, New South Wales: Random House, 1993), 172–178, 233–253.

263   J. Longman, "An Amputee Sprinter: Is He Disabled or Too-Abled?" *The New York Times*, May 15, 2007, http://1ref.us/9u (accessed April 27, 2015); D. Snowdon, *Aging with Grace* (London: Fourth Estate, 2001), 117, 118.

264   M. J. Valenzuela, *Maintain Your Brain* (Australia: HarperCollins Publishers, 2011).

265   Shaffer, *Personality Development*, 356.

Chapter 5

266   E. A. Laws, *Aquatic Pollution* (New York: John Wiley & Sons, Inc., 1993), 356–396, 495, 496.

267   F. Baum, *The New Public Health*, 2nd ed. (Oxford: Oxford University Press, 2002), 267–270; R. Bertollini et al., eds., *Environmental Epidemiology: Exposure and Disease* (New York: Lewis Publishers, 1996), 11, 12, 148–154, 167–172; Finkelstein et al., *American Journal of Epidemiology* 160 (2004): 173–177; H. Warwick, *New Scientist* 180, no. 2424 (2003): 22; J-P. Zock et al., *American Journal of Respiratory and Critical Care Medicine* 163, no. 7 (2001): 1572–1577.

268   Kumar et al., *Robbins Basic Pathology*, 281–286.

269   G. R. Conway and J. N. Pretty, *Unwelcome Harvest: Agriculture and Pollution* (London: Earthscan Publications Ltd, 1991), 251–261; L. Fewtrell, *Environmental Health Perspectives* 112, no. 4 (2004): 1371–1374.

270   G. J. Tortora et al., *Microbiology: An Introduction*, 6th ed. (Menlo Park, CA: Addison Wesley Longman, Inc., 1998), 413; D. A. Walton et al., *New England Journal of Medicine* 364, no. 1 (2011): 3–5.

271   23rd Australian Total Diet Study, http://1ref.us/9v (accessed April 27, 2015).

272   R. Ghandhi and S. Snedeker, "Pesticide Residue Monitoring and Food Safety," Cornell University Program on Breast Cancer and Environmental Risk Factors in New York State, Fact sheet no. 25, 1999, http://1ref.us/9w (accessed February 10, 2015); L. Karalliedde et al., *Organophosphates and Health* (London: Imperial College Press, 2001), 252–454.

273   N. Y. Dionson, *ACIAR Newsletter*, no. 36 (April–September) (2000): 11; M. Rechcigl, ed., *CRC Handbook Series in Nutrition and Food*, section E (West Palm Beach, FL: CRC Press, 1978), 2, 215–220.

274   Bertollini et al., *Environmental Epidemiology*, 10–12; F. Perera et al., *Environmental Research* 114 (2012): 40–46.

275   A. Gosline, *New Scientist* 183, no. 2454 (2004): 14; I. N. Krivoshto et al., *Journal of the American Board of Family Medicine* 21, no. 1 (2008): 55–62.

276   F. Pearce and R. Edwards, *New Scientist* 175, no. 2356 (2002): 8, 9; P. J. Sheehan et al., eds., *Effects of Pollutants at the Ecosystem Level* (New York: John Wiley & Sons Ltd, 1984), 195–237; World Health Organization, "Ambient (Outdoor) Air Quality and Health," http://1ref.us/9x (accessed February 10, 2015).

277   Laws, *Aquatic Pollution*, 75, 76; Pacific Institute, "World Water Quality Facts and Statistics," http://1ref.us/9y (accessed April 27, 2015).

278   G. E. Greening, *Microbiology Australia* 34, no. 2 (2013): 63–66; J. M. H. Selendy, ed., *Water and Sanitation Related Diseases and the Environment* (New York: John Wiley & Sons, 2011), 271–288; R. J. Wittman and G. J. Flick, *Annual Review of Public Health* 16 (1995): 123–140.

279   Baum, *New Public Health*, 434–436; C. F. Graumann and S. Moscovici, eds., *Changing Conceptions of Crowd Mind and Behaviour* (New York: Springer-Verlag, 1986), 134–139; K. Wolf and K. Flora, "Mental Health and Function," http://1ref.us/9z (accessed February 10, 2015).

280   Baum, *New Public Health*, 434; Graumann & Moscovici, *Changing Conceptions*, 118–120.

281   D. Clarke, *Pro-social and Anti-social Behaviour* (New York: Routledge, 2003), 79–98; Graumann & Moscovici, *Changing Conceptions*, 11–15.

282   Rice, *The Adolescent*, 410–414.

283   Institute of Medicine (US), *Damp Indoor Spaces and Health* (Washington, DC: National Academies Press, 2004), 146–149; W. A. Shipton, *The Biology of Fungi Impacting Human Health* (Singapore: Trafford Publishing, 2013), 33; S. J. Vesper et al., *Applied and Environmental Microbiology* 65 (1999): 3175–3181.

284   B. Richardson, *Wood Preservation* (New York: Taylor & Francis, 1993), 122.

285   Y. Assouline-Dayan et al., *Journal of Asthma* 39 (2002): 191–201; Institute of Medicine (US), *Damp Indoor Spaces*, 170, 171.

286   Bertollini, *Environmental Epidemiology*, 167–174.

287   L. Gari, "Ecology in Muslim Heritage: Treatises on Environmental Pollution up to the End of the 13th Century," http://1ref.us/a0 (accessed February 10, 2015).

288   D. Urbinato, "London's Historic 'Pea-Soupers,'" *EPA Journal* (Summer 1994): http://1ref.us/a1 (accessed February 10, 2015).

289   Richard Bauckham, "Reading the Bible in the Context of the Ecological Threats of Our Time," 64th Annual Meeting of the Evangelical Theological Society, "Caring for Creation," November 14–16, 2012, Milwaukee, Wis.

290   It often is argued that the later text does not apply primarily to activities involving destruction of the biosphere,

but speaks of judgments on parties and individuals on account of their moral wickedness. Ultimately, however, moral decline impacts the environment (2 Samuel 12:9–18; Hosea 4:1–10). Lack of stewardship on one area is followed by neglect in others.

291   Genisis 2:2; W. A. Shipton, *The Golden River That Flows Through Time* (Tamarac, FL: Llumina Press, 2010), 152.

292   Romans 1:20; W. A. Shipton, *Asia-Africa Journal of Mission and Ministry* 4 (2011): 135–154.

293   A. P. Wolf and W. H. Durham, *Inbreeding, Incest and the Incest Taboo: The State of Knowledge at the Turn of the Century* (Stanford, CA: Stanford University Press, 2004), 49–54.

294   R. A. Busuttil et al., *PLOS One* 2, no. 9 (2007): e876, doi:10.1371/journal.pone.0000876; H-C. Lee and Y-H. Wei, *Experimental Biology and Medicine* 232 (2007): 592–606.

295   Example: K. Christensen et al., *Nature Reviews* 7 (2006): 436–448.

296   Compare with animal studies—R. Frankham, *Heredity* 78, no. 3 (1977): 311–327; M. D. B. Eldridge et al., *Conservation Biology* 13, no. 3 (1999): 531–541.

297   J. Charrow, *Familial Cancer* 3 (2004): 201–206; H. Chen and A. Laufer-Cahana, *eMedicine*, November 6 (2007), http://1ref.us/a2 (accessed February 10, 2015); V. A. McKusick et al., *Cold Spring Harbor Symposia on Quantitative Biology* 29 (1964): 99–114; L. B. Weinstein, *Family and Community Health* 30, no. 1 (2007): 50–62; T-L. Young et al., *American Journal of Human Genetics* 65 (1999): 1680–1687.

298   G. F. Stine, *Biogenetics: Human Heredity and Social Issues* (New York: Macmillan Publishing Company, Inc., 1977), 388.

299   Y. Ghodke et al., *European Journal of Epidemiology* 20 (2005): 475–488; Weinstein, *Family and Community Health* (2007); A. G. White et al., *British Journal of Ophthalmology* 81 (1997): 431–434; A. F. Wright and N. Hastie, *Genes and Common Diseases: Genetics in Modern Medicine* (Cambridge: Cambridge University Press, 2007), 142–271.

300   Example: myxomatosis in rabbits and malaria in humans—L. H. **Miller,** *Proceedings of the National Academy of Sciences USA* 91, no. 7 (**1994**): 2415–2419; C. K. Williams et al., *Australian Journal of Zoology* **38** (1990): 697–703.

301   Ghodke et al., *European Journal of Epidemiology* (2005); Weinstein, *Family and Community Health* (2007); White et al., *British Journal of Ophthalmology* (1997); Wright & Hastie, *Genes and Common Diseases*, 142–271.

302   S. J. O'Brien et al., *Science* 227 (1985): 1428–1434.

303   M. E. Jones et al., *Proceedings of the National Academy of Sciences USA* 105, no. 20 (2008): 10023–10027; K. B. Wyatt et al., *PLOS One* 3, no. 11 (2008): e3602, doi:10.1371/journal.pone.0003602.

304   D. Pimentel, ed., *Encyclopedia of Pest Management* (New York: Marcel Dekker, Inc., 2002), 162–164.

305   This is seen after a number of texts are examined—human activities are destroying the earth (Revelation 11:18); ecological disasters can be due to environmental extremes, human

extravagance, and neglect (1 Kings 17:1, 7; 18:41–44; Proverbs 24:30, 31; Ezekiel 14:13; Amos 4:6–9); ecological recovery is possible (Ezekiel 47:1–10), some animals require special habitats (Job 39:5–8); resources are to be used judiciously (Numbers 11:31–34; Isaiah 9:9–11); nature is God's second book of information about His character that should not be neglected (Psalm 19:4; Romans 1:20); and all our activities are to bring glory to God (1 Corinthians 10:31).

306 Sandra Richter, "Environmental Law: Wisdom from the Ancients," 64th Annual Meeting of the Evangelical Theological Society, "Caring for Creation," November 14–16, 2012, Milwaukee, Wis.

307 The instructions given by God to Noah on the arrangements for the continuation of various animal kinds after the flood can be taken as indicating the preservation priorities we might follow today.

308 H. Büssow, *The Quest for Food* (New York: Springer Science+Business Media, LLC, 2007), 639–647; K. V. Krishnamurthy, *Textbook of Biodiversity* (Enfield, NH: Science Publishers, Inc., 2003), 47–50.

309 Romans 1:20; Shipton, *Golden River*, 152–156.

310 L. E. Datnoff et al., eds., *Mineral Nutrition and Plant Disease* (St Paul, MN: APS Press, 2007); T. M. Spann and A. W. Shcumann, "Mineral Nutrition Contributes to Plant Disease and Pest Resistance," University of Florida IFAS Extension, publication HS1181 (2013), http://1ref.us/a3 (accessed February 10, 2015).

311 D. M. Rohl, *A Test of Time. The Bible—from Myth to History* (London: Century, 1995), 1: 282.

312 Bryan, *Food, Nutrition*, 36, 69, 72, 87, 92, 98, 162.

313 G. J. Wenham, *The Book of Leviticus. The New International Commentary on the Old Testament* (Grand Rapids, MI: William B. Eerdmans Publishing Company, 1979), 211, 212.

314 R. N. Bellah et al., *Habits of the Heart* (Berkeley, CA: University of California Press, 1985), 276, 277.

315 J. Stevenson, *The Complete Idiot's Guide to Philosophy*, 3rd ed. (New York: Alpha Books, 2005), 31–35.

316 A. Oliver, *Institute for Christian Teaching* 24CC (1999): 217–236.

317 D. Kellner, *Jean Baudrillard: From Marxism to Postmodernism and Beyond* (Cambridge: Polity Press, 1989), 93–121.

318 J. Ridgeway, *Middle States Geographer* 41 (2008): 45–52.

319 R. S. White, ed., *Creation in Crisis: Christian Perspectives on Sustainability* (London: SPCK, 2009), 241–254.

320 E. Aagaard, *Adventists Affirm* 16, no. 1 (2002): 33–40; M. Behe, *Darwin's Black Box: The Biochemical Challenge to Evolution* (New York: The Free Press, 1996).

321 D. L. Hull, *Nature* 352 (1991): 485, 486.

Chapter 6

322 Bryan, *Food, Nutrition*; E. A. Noyes, *Spiritualistic Deceptions in Health and Healing* (Monrovia, CA: Homeward Publishing, 2007), 73–129; D. R. Varma,

The Art and Science of Healing Since Antiquity (Bloomington, IN: Xlibris Corporation, 2011), 186–189.

323   J. G. Black, *Microbiology: Principles and Explorations*, 6th ed. (Hoboken, NJ: John Wiley & Sons, Inc., 2005), 11–14.

324   B. Hampil, *Journal of Bacteriology* 16, no. 5 (1928): 287–300; E. W. Nester et al., *Microbiology: A Human Perspective*, 4th ed. (New York: McGraw-Hill, 2004), 489, 490.

325   J. M. McCulloch and L. C. Kloth, *Wound Healing*, 4th ed. (Philadelphia: F. A. Davis Company, 2010), 576, 577.

326   B. Brier and H. Hobbs, *Daily Life of the Ancient Egyptians*, 2nd ed. (Westport, CT: Greenwood Press, 2008), 271–273; J. P. Byrne, ed., *Encyclopedia of Pestilence, Pandemics, and Plagues* (Westport, CT: Greenwood Press, 2008), 1: 357; D. R. Hopkins, *The Greatest Killer: Smallpox in History* (Chicago: University of Chicago Press, 2002), 14–16, 20; J. F. Nunn, *Ancient Egyptian Medicine* (Norman, OK: University of Oklahoma Press, 2002), 96.

327   Hopkins, *Greatest Killer*, 14–16, 20; Rohl, *Test of Time*, 1, 280.

328   S. T. Peters, *Epidemic: Smallpox in the New World* (New York: Benchmark Books, 2005), 4, 5.

329   A. L. Melnick, *Biological, Chemical, and Radiological Terrorism* (New York: Springer Science+Business Media, LLC, 2008), 41–43.

330   R. M. Bhat and C. Prakash, *Interdisciplinary Perspectives on Infectious Diseases* (2012); article ID 181089, http://1ref.us/a4 (accessed April 27, 2015); B. K. Girdhar, *Indian Journal of Dermatology, Venereology and Leprology* 71, no. 4 (2005): 223–225; M. Lavania et al., *Infection, Genetics and Evolution* 8, no. 5 (2008): 627–631.

331   M. Tajkarimi et al., *Trends in Food Science & Technology* 29, no. 2 (2013): 116–123.

332   I. Singer et al., eds., "Ablution," *The Jewish Encyclopedia* (New York: Funk & Wagnalls, 1906), http://1ref.us/a5 (accessed February 10, 2015).

333   M. Asktar, "Public Health Aspects of the House Fly, *Musca domestica* L. (Diptera: Muscidae)—*Enterococcus* spp." (PhD diss., Kansas State University, 2008), 7, 8.

334   M. Förster et al., *Veterinary Parasitology* 160, no. 1–2 (2009): 163–167; V. J. Fraser et al., *Diseases and Disorders* (New York: Marshall Cavendish, 2008), 3: 744–747; D. T. Jamison et al., eds., *Disease Control Priorities in Developing Countries*, 2nd ed. (New York: Oxford University Press, 2006), 24: 16, doi:10.1596/978-0-821-36179-5/Chpt-24.

335   J. Fawell and M. J. Nieuwenhuijsen, *British Medical Bulletin* 68, no. 1 (2003): 199–208.

336   J. A. Romano et al., eds., *Chemical Warfare Agents: Chemistry, Pharmacology, Toxicology, and Therapeutics*, 2nd ed. (Boca Raton, FL: CRC Group, 2008), 53.

337   A. Dufour et al., eds., *Animal Waste, Water Quality and Human Health* (London: IWA Publishing, 2012), 75–95.

338   S. J. Olsen et al., *Emerging Infectious Diseases* 8, no. 4 (2002): 370–375.

339   B. S. Levy and V. W. Sidel, *Social Injustice*

and *Public Health* (Oxford: Oxford University Press, 2005), 226.

340   L. Hardinge, *With Jesus in His Sanctuary* (Harrisburg, PA: American Cassette Ministries, 1991), 389, 390.

341   A. Davies and R. Board, eds., *The Microbiology of Meat and Poultry* (London: Blackie Academic & Professional, 1998), 238.

342   A. Beetz, ed., *Bestiality and Zoophilia. Sexual Relationships with Animals* (West Lafayette, IN: Purdue University Press, 2005), 1–22, 98–119; F. A. Schaeffer, *How Should We Then Live?* (Old Tappan, NJ: Fleming H. Revell Company, 1976), 24–29.

343   M. D. R. Evans and J. Kelley, *Religion, Morality and Public Policy in International Perspective, 1984–2002* (Annandale, New South Wales: Federation Press, 2002), 89, 90.

344   F. L. de Melo et al., *PLOS Neglected Tropical Diseases* 4, no. 1 (2010): e575, http://1ref.us/a6 (accessed February 10, 2015); B. M. Rothschild, *Clinical Infectious Diseases* 40 (2005): 1454–1463.

345   S. Loue, ed., *Mental Health Practitioner's Guide to HIV/AIDS* (New York: Springer Science+Business Media, 2013), 155–157.

346   P. J. Bomar, ed., *Promoting Health in Families*, 3rd ed. (Philadelphia: Saunders, 2004), 434; F. E. Fox and D. W. Virtue, *Homosexuality: Good & Right in the Eyes of God*, 2nd ed. (Alexandria, VA: Emmaus Ministries, 2003), 240.

347   Nester, et al., *Microbiology*, 492.

348   S. H. Horn, *Seventh-day Adventist Bible Dictionary* (Washington, DC: Review and Herald Publishing Association, 1960), 8–11, 99, 100, 103–105, 737–742 on the topics of Abraham and Moses with A. P. Wolf and W. H. Durham, *Inbreeding, Incest and the Incest Taboo: The State of Knowledge at the Turn of the Century* (Stanford, CA: Stanford University Press, 2004), 49–54.

349   R. A. Busuttil et al., *PLOS One* 2, no. 9 (2007): e876, doi:10.1371/journal.pone.0000876; Lee and Wei, *Experimental Biology and Medicine* (2007).

350   Example: K. Christensen et al., *Nature Reviews* 7 (2006): 436–448.

351   A. Trifunovic et al, *Nature* 429 (2004): 417–423.

352   Compare with animal studies—M. D. B. Eldridge et al., *Conservation Biology* 13, no. 3 (1999): 531–541; R. Frankham, *Heredity* 78, no. 3 (1997): 311–327.

353   J. Charrow, *Familial Cancer* 3 (2004): 201–206; Chen and Laufer-Cahana, *eMedicine* (2007); McKusick et al., *Cold Spring Harbor Symposia on Quantitative Biology* (1964); Weinstein, *Family and Community Health* (2007); Young *et al. American Journal of Human Genetics* (1999).

354   Stine, *Biogenetics*, 388.

355   A. Christianson et al., *Global Report on Birth Defects* (New York: March of Dimes Birth Defects Foundation, 2006), 21, 22; H. Hamamy, *Journal of Community Genetics* 3, no. 3 (2012): 185–192.

356   E. Cockburn and T. A. Reyman, eds., *Mummies, Disease & Ancient Cultures*, 2nd ed. (Cambridge: Cambridge University Press, 1998), 38–58.

357   Molly Billings, "The influenza Pandemic of 1918," June 1997, modified February 2005, http://1ref.us/a7 (accessed February 10, 2015); N. D. Cook, *Born to Die: Disease and New World Conquest* (Cambridge: University of Cambridge Press, 1998), 86–165; K. Cunningham, *The Bubonic Plague* (Edina, MN: ABDO Publishing Company, 2011), 34–81; Madigan et al., *Brock Biology* (2003), 858–860, 892, 926.

358   Examples: myxomatosis in rabbits and malaria in humans—L. H. Miller, *Proceedings of the National Academy of Science USA* 91, no. 7 (1994): 2415–2419; C. K. Williams et al., *Australian Journal of Zoology* 38 (1990): 697–703.

359   D. P. Kwiatkowski, *American Journal of Human Genetics* 77 (2005): 171–192.

360   S. Moalem, *New Scientist* 193, no. 2591 (2007): 42–45.

361   Y. Ghodke et al., *European Journal of Epidemiology* 20 (2005): 475–488; Weinstein, *Family and Community Health* (2007); A. G. White et al., *British Journal of Ophthalmology* 81 (1997): 431–434; A. F. Wright and N. Hastie, *Genes and Common Diseases: Genetics in Modern Medicine* (Cambridge: Cambridge University Press, 2007), 142–271.

362   M. E. Jones et al., *Proceedings of the National Academy of Sciences USA* 105, no. 20 (2008): 10023–10027; O'Brien et al., *Science* (1985); K. B. Wyatt et al., *PLOS One* 3, no. 11 (2008): e3602, doi:10.1371/journal.pone.0003602.

363   L. V. Marks and M. P. Worboys, eds., *Migrants, Minorities and Health* (London: Routledge, 1997), 193–195.

364   Ibid., 194, 207.

365   P. K. Drain et al., *BMC Infectious Diseases* 6 (2006): 172, doi:10.1186/1471-2334-6-172; H. A. Weiss et al., *Sexually Transmitted Infections* 82, no. 2 (2006): 101–109.

366   H. G. Koenig et al., *Handbook of Religion and Health*, 2nd ed. (Oxford: Oxford University Press, 2012), 224–235, 450–467.

367   G. Legood, ed., *Veterinary Ethics: An Introduction* (London: Continuum International Publishing Group, 2000), 115.

368   T. R. Rich, "Kashrut: Jewish Dietary Laws," http://1ref.us/a8 (accessed February 10, 2015).

369   M. Tajkarimi et al., *Trends in Food Science & Technology* 29, no. 2 (2013): 116–123.

370   I. Guerrero-Legarreta, ed., *Handbook of Poultry Science and Technology: Secondary Processing* (Hoboken, NJ: John Wiley & Sons, Inc., 2010), 2: 393.

371   D. Shin et al., *Poultry Science* 91, no. 12 (2012): 3247–3252.

372   M. N. Hajmeer et al., *Journal of Food Science* 64, no. 4 (1999): 719–723.

373   A. Green, *Field Guide to Meat: How to Identify, Select, and Prepare Virtually Every Meat, Poultry, and Game Cut* (Philadelphia: Quirk Books, 2005), 3.

Section II: Mental and Social Health

374   Quote Garden, http://1ref.us/8n (accessed June 3, 2015); Brainy Quotes, http://1ref.us/8k (accessed June 3, 2015); The Virtual Library of Public Health, http://1ref.us/a9 (accessed June 3, 2015).

Chapter 7

375 D. Comeau, *EGallery* 8, no. 3 (2002), http://1ref.us/az (accessed June 8, 2015).

376 W. D. Wall, *Education and Mental Health*, 2nd ed. (London: George G. Harrap & Co. Ltd, 1956), preface, 17.

377 Ibid., 20–27.

378 B. L. Reece and B. Brandt, *Effective Human Relations: Personal and Organizational Applications*, 8th ed. (Boston: Houghton Mifflin Company, 2002), 146–150.

379 J. Cohen, ed., *Educating Hearts and Minds* (New York: Teachers College Press, 1999), 10, 11; K. Weare, *Promoting Mental, Emotional and Social Health* (London: Routledge, 2000), 11.

380 D. Goleman, *Emotional Intelligence* (London: Bloomsbury Publishing, 1996), 8, 9, 36, 42, 43.

381 Ibid., 43–53, 56–58, 78–89; Weare, *Promoting Mental … Health*, 63.

382 Rice, *The Adolescent*, 174–176.

383 A. Nygren, *Agape and Eros*, trans. P. S. Watson (Chicago: University of Chicago Press, 1982), 77, 78; White, *The Desire of Ages*, 667, 668.

384 R. W. Wolfe and C. E. Gudorf, eds., *Ethics and World Religions* (Marynoll, NY: Orbis Books, 1999), 368–373.

385 C. S. Lewis, *The Abolition of Man* (New York: Macmillan Publishing Co., Inc., 1973), 95–121.

386 D. K. Nelson, *Outrageous Grace* (Nampa, ID: Pacific Press Publishing Association, 1998), 44, 45.

387 McMillen & Stern, *None of These Diseases*, 207–210.

388 T. Buckley et al., *European Heart Journal, Acute Cardiovascular Care* (February 23, 2015): doi:10.1177/2048872615568969.

389 Goleman, *Emotional Intelligence*, 86, 87.

390 J. R. Durant, ed., *Human Origins* (Oxford: Clarendon Press, 1989), 137–143; S. Hawking, *A Brief History of Time* (New York: Bantam Books, 1988), 122–141, 175.

391 S. J. Lopez, ed., *Positive Psychology: Discovering Human Strengths* (Westport, CT: Greenwood Publishing Group, Inc., 2008), 131–149; Seligman, *Learned Optimism*, 171–174.

392 Goleman, *Emotional Intelligence*, 96, 97, 104–106.

393 J. Delumeau, *Sin and Fear* (New York: St. Martin's Press, 1990), 373–382, 536–554; J. Le Goff, *The Birth of Purgatory* (London: Scolar Press, 1984), 52, 53; O. Pfister, *Christianity and Fear* (London: George Allen & Unwin Ltd, 1948), 155, 157; the words translated in most texts as "hell" might also legitimately be translated as "the place of the dead"—A. Cruden, *Cruden's Complete Concordance to the Old and New Testament* (London: Lutterworth Press, 1958), 297.

394 Goleman, *Emotional Intelligence*, 113–119.

395 L. Dunstan, *Signs of the Times* 117, no. 11 (2002): 32–36.

396 K. L. Jones et al., *Emotional Health*, 2nd ed. (San Francisco: Canfield Press, 1975), 8, 9.

397 Weare, *Promoting Mental … Health*, 5.

398 Ibid., 14–16.

399 J. Fabian, *Creative Thinking and Problem Solving* (Chelsea, MI: Lewis Publishers, 1990), 6–10.

400   Dunstan, *Signs of the Times* (2002).

401   J. McDowell, *Evidence that Demands a Verdict*, revised edition (San Bernardino, CA: Here's Life Publishers, Inc., 1979), 166–175, 267–320.

402   I. Berczi and A. Szentivanyi, eds., *Neuroimmune Biology* (Amsterdam: Elsevier, 2001), 1: 351–364; C. Magai and S. H. McFadden, eds., *Handbook of Emotion, Adult Development, and Aging* (London: Academic Press, 1996), 309, 310; Seligman, *Learned Optimism*, 172–174.

403   M. A. Smialek, *Team Strategies for Success* (Lanham, MD: The Scarecrow Press, Inc., 2001), 5, 6.

404   Rushton, *Altruism*, 170–173.

405   Bellah et al., *Habits of the Heart*, 142–144, 276–282; P. Ustinov, *Ustinov Still at Large* (London: Michael O'Mara Books Limited, 1993), 137–139.

406   C. E. Izard, *The Psychology of Emotions* (New York: Plenum Press, 1991), 205–226; J. F. Sowislo and U. Orth, *Psychological Bulletin 139* (2013): 213–240.

407   Magai and McFadden, *Handbook of Emotion*, 308, 309.

408   B. L. Beezold et al., *Nutrition Journal* (2010): 9: 26, doi:10.1186/1475-2891-9-26.

409   Shaffer, *Personality Development*, 384, 387–390.

410   Nygren, *Agape and Eros*, 214–219.

Chapter 8

411   J. S. Hyde, *American Psychologist* 60, no. 6 (2005): 581–592; G. Reevy et al., *Encyclopedia of Emotion* (Santa Barbara, CA: ABC-CLIO, LLC, 2010), 283–285; R. K. Unger, ed., *Handbook of the Psychology of Women and Gender* (Hoboken, NJ: John Wiley & Sons, Inc., 2004), 245–255.

412   M. Eastman, *Family: The Vital Factor* (Melbourne: Collins Dove, 1989), 159–176.

413   A. E. Gottfried and A. W. Gottfried, eds., *Redefining Families: Implications for Children's Development* (New York: Plenum Press, 1994), 3–6; D. Popenoe, *War Over the Family* (New Brunswick, NJ: Transaction Publishers, 2008), 3–41.

414   Eastman, *Family*, 3, 4.

415   M. Bloom, *Primary Prevention Practices* (Thousand Oakes, CA: Sage Publications, Inc., 1996), 192–195; Eastman, *Family*, 4–12.

416   D. Coon and J. O. Mitterer, *Introduction to Psychology: Gateways to Mind and Behavior*, 12th ed. (Melbourne: Cengage Learning, 2008), 92.

417   Eastman, *Family*, 11–19; A. West and H. Pennell, *Underachievement in Schools* (London: RoutledgeFalmer, 2003), 47–49.

418   Eastman, *Family*, 21–37, 63–88; Z. Merali, *New Scientist* 193, no. 2587 (2007): 8.

419   Eastman, *Family*, 68.

420   Clark, *Paediatrics & Child Health* 18, no. 7 (2013): 373–377; Eastman, *Family*, 68; S. Goldstein and R. B. Brooks, eds., *Handbook of Resilience in Children*, 2nd ed. (New York: Springer Science+Business Media, 2013), 448, 449; H. I. McCubbin et al., eds., *The*

Dynamics of Resilient Families (London: Sage Publications, 1999), 6.

421 V. L. Bengtson et al., *How Families Still Matter* (Cambridge: Cambridge University Press, 2003), 90.

422 Eastman, *Family*, 72, 73; Weare, *Promoting Mental … Health*, 24, 64–65.

423 A. B. David, *Around the Shabbat Table: A Guide to Fulfilling and Meaningful Shabbat Table Conversations* (Northvale, NJ: Jason Aronson, 2000), 60, 61.

424 Eastman, *Family*, 66, 67; Goldstein and Brooks, *Handbook of Resilience*, 446–455.

425 Goldstein and Brooks, *Handbook of Resilience*, 453, 454; Seligman, *Learned Optimism*, 233–253.

426 J. M. Lewis et al., *No Single Thread* (New York: Brunner/Mazel, Publishers, 1976), 210; Shaffer, *Personality Development*, 430–432.

427 Eastman, *Family*, 74–80; Shaffer, *Personality Development*, 222–225, 453–458.

428 Q. N. Lee-Chua, *Successful Family Businesses* (Manila: Ateneo de Manila University Press, 2003), 28, 29; Popenoe, *War Over the Family*, 46–52.

429 F. Coakey, "Dorcas Society," http://1ref.us/ab (accessed February 10, 2015).

430 Autism Society of America, http://1ref.us/ac (accessed June 4, 2015); Breast Cancer Society of Canada, http://1ref.us/ad (accessed June 4, 2015); Leukemia and Lymphoma Society, http://1ref.us/ae (accessed June 4, 2015).

431 Rushton, *Altruism*, 170–175.

432 E. Roos et al., *Public Health Nutrition* 17,

no. 11 (2014): 2528–2536, doi:10.1017/S1368980013002954.

433 D. Petre, *Father Time* (Sydney: Pan Macmillan Australia, 1998), 61–69.

434 Goldstein and Brooks, *Handbook of Resilience*, 449, 450.

435 Eastman, *Family*, 83, 84.

436 Lewis et al., *No Single Thread*, 102, 209–211, 222–224.

437 Magai & McFadden, *Handbook of Emotion,* 351–356.

438 W. Shipton et al., *Worldviews and Christian Education* (Singapore: Trafford Publishing, 2013), 336–342; 572–578.

439 R. A. Emmons, *Journal of Personality and Social Psychology* 84, no. 2 (2003): 377–389.

440 Shaffer, *Personality Development*, 427–433.

441 A. Campbell et al., "Polygamy in Canada: Legal and Social Implications for Women and Children—A Collection of Policy Research Reports" (2005), http://1ref.us/af (accessed February 10, 2015); T. Griffith, ed., *The Travels of Marco Polo* (Hertfordshire, UK: Wordsworth Editions Limited, 1997), 62, 63, 73, 95–96; IslamReligion.com, "An Introduction to Polygamy within Islam" (2006), http://1ref.us/ag (accessed February 10, 2015).

442 R. Du Preez, *Journal of the Adventist Theological Society* 10, no. 1–2 (1999): 33–39.

443 Popenoe, *War Over the Family*, 49, 56, 57.

444 J. B. Benson and M. M. Haith, *Social and Emotional Development in Infancy and Early Childhood* (San Diego, CA,

Elsevier, Inc., 2009), 280–292; Coon and Mitterer, *Introduction to Psychology*, 91, 92.

445   Eastman, *Family*, 186–190.

446   Benson and Haith, *Social and Emotional Development*, 142, 143.

447   Ibid., 143; Shaffer, *Personality Development*, 427–433.

Chapter 9

448   Bellah et al., *Habits of the Heart*, 142–151.

449   P. Dickens, *Social Darwinism* (Buckingham: The Open University Press, 2000), 80–84, 101–109.

450   Bellah et al., *Habits of the Heart*, 116–118.

451   Ibid., 155–160.

452   R. Lacayo and A. Ripley, *Time*, Australia, December 30–January 6 (2002/2003), 34.

453   Bellah et al., *Habits of the Heart*, 159–162, 196–198.

454   United Nations, "Universal Declaration of Human Rights," http://1ref.us/ah (accessed April 27, 2015).

455   Nygren, *Agape and Eros*, 78.

456   E. G. White, *Mind, Character, and Personality* (Nashville: Southern Publishing Association, 1977), 1: 259–262.

457   S. Roffey, ed., *Positive Relationships; Evidence Based Practice across the World* (New York: Springer Science+Business Media B. V., 2005), 93, 94; Shaffer, *Personality Development*, 222–225.

458   Shaffer, *Personality Development*, 346–349.

459   R. C. Beck, *Motivation: Theories and Principles* (Upper Saddle River, NJ: Prentice Hall, 2000), 315.

460   Rushton, *Altruism*, 3, 4.

461   R. Gilman et al., eds., *Handbook of Psychology in Schools* (New York: Routledge, 2009), 122–124; Shaffer, *Personality Development*, 364–369.

462   Gilman et al., *Handbook of Psychology*, 122, 123; Shaffer, *Personality Development*, 373, 376.

463   Gilman et al., *Handbook of Psychology*, 123; Shaffer, *Personality Development*, 392, 393.

464   Gilman et al., *Handbook of Psychology*, 123.

465   Rushton, *Altruism*, 115–126, 133–155; Shaffer, *Personality Development*, 282–285, 356, 387–392.

466   Rushton, *Altruism*, 81–85, 121.

467   Ibid., 387, 388.

468   Popenoe, *War Over the Family*, 46–57.

469   N. M. Hurd et al., *Journal of Youth and Adolescence* 38, no. 6 (2010): 777–789.

470   Popenoe, *War Over the Family*, 149, 150; Shaffer, *Personality Development*, 346–351.

471   Anderson et al., *Psychological Bulletin* (2010); E. Gullone, *Animal Cruelty, Antisocial Behaviour, and Aggression: More than a Link* (New York: Palgrave Macmillan, 2012), 60–62; Rushton, *Altruism*, 135–144.

472   S. L. Douglass and M. A. Shaikh, *Current Issues in Comparative Education* 7, no. 1 (2004): 5–18.

473   W. Richey, "U.S. Supreme Court Takes a New 10 Commandments Case," April 1,

2008, http://1ref.us/ai (accessed February 10, 2015); Rushton, *Altruism*, 170–177; BBC News. "US Bans Commandments in Courtroom," March 3, 2005, http://1ref.us/aj (accessed April 28, 2015).

474   A. Lindsley, *C. S. Lewis's Case for Christ: Insights from Reason, Imagination, and Faith* (Nottingham, UK: InterVarsity Press, 2005), 155.

475   Office of the Education Council, *Education in Thailand 2007* (Bangkok: Amarin, 2008), 178–182.

476   W. B. Russell and S. Waters, *Reel Character Education: A Cinematic Approach to Character Development* (Charlotte, NC: IAP-Information Age Publishing, Inc., 2010), 11–18.

477   J. Arthur, *Education with Character: The Moral Economy of Schooling* (New York: RoutledgeFalmer, 2003), 50–57; G. R. Knight, *Journal of Adventist Education* (Summer 2005): 6–9.

478   D. Underwood, *From Yahweh to Yahoo! The Religious Roots of the Secular Press* (Champaign, IL: University of Illinois Press, 2008), 149–152.

Chapter 10

479   P. Dewe et al., *Coping with Work Stress: A Review and Critique* (Chichester, West Sussex: John Wiley & Sons, Ltd, 2010), 2–6.

480   N. A. Campbell et al., *Essential Biology with Physiology* (San Francisco: Benjamin Cummings, 2004), 553–555; L. Sherwood, *Human Physiology: From Cells to Systems*, 7th ed. (Belmont, CA: Brooks/Cole, Cengage Learning, 2010), 700–710.

481   McMillen and Stern, *None of These Diseases*, 175–177; C. Starr and B. McMillan, *Human Biology*, 8th ed. (Belmont, CA: Brooks/Cole, Cengage Learning, 2010), 296, 297; Zacharias, *Mediterranean Diet*, 29–33.

482   F. Toates, *Stress: Conceptual and Biological Aspects* (Chichester: John Wiley and Sons, 1995), 252–254.

483   Seaward, *Managing Stress*, 108–120; L. Steinberg et al., *Life-span Development: Infancy through Adulthood* (Belmont, CA: Wadsworth, Cengage Learning, 2011), 489; Toates, *Stress*, 254–256.

484   T. M. Bayless and A. Diehl, eds., *Advanced Therapy in Gastroenterology and Liver Disease*, 5th ed. (Hamilton, Ontario: BC Decker, Inc., 2005), 260.

485   R. S. Irwin and J. M. Rippe, eds., *Irwin and Rippe's Intensive Care Medicine* (Philadelphia: Lippincott Williams & Wilkins, 2008), 1181, 1182; Toates, *Stress*, 275, 277.

486   R. Ader, ed., *Psychoneuroimmunology*, 4th ed. (Burlington, MD: Elsevier Academic Press, 2007), 881, 882; A. Conti, *New York Academy of Sciences* 917 (2000): 68–83; R. J. Contrada and A. Baum, eds., *The Handbook of Stress Science: Biology, Psychology, and Health* (New York: Springer Publishing Company, LLC, 2011), 421; Toates, *Stress*, 261–263.

487   J. Giorando and J. Engebretson, *Explore (NY)* 2 (2006): 216–225; Magai and McFadden, *Handbook of Emotion*, 351–359; Seaward, *Managing Stress*, 128–155.

488   Seaward, *Managing Stress*, 163–165.

489   A. Carr, *Positive Psychology: The Science of Happiness and Human Strengths*

(New York: Routledge, 2004), 216, 217; Contrada and Baum, *Handbook of Stress*, 223, 225.

490   H. S. Friedman, ed., *The Oxford Handbook of Health Psychology* (New York: Oxford University Press, Inc., 2011), 167–170.

491   Contrada and Baum, *Handbook of Stress*, 223; Seaward, *Managing Stress*, 176, 190, 204, 217, 235, 251, 263, 278, 292, 322, 369, 386.

492   Seaward, *Managing Stress*, 169–173.

493   Ibid., 172–175.

494   D. Frownfelter and E. Dean, *Cardiovascular and Pulmonary Physical Therapy: Evidence to Practice*, 5th ed. (St Louis, MO: Elsevier Mosby, 2012), 9.

495   Ibid., 182–184.

496   Rohl, *Test of Time*, 1: 327–367.

497   Carr, *Positive Psychology*, 218.

498   Seaward, *Managing Stress*, 239–251.

499   Ibid., 253–263.

500   W. Whiston, trans., *The Life and Works of Flavius Josephus. Antiquities of the Jews* (Philadelphia: The John C Winston Company, c. 1936), 92, 93.

501   Seaward, *Managing Stress*, 271–274.

502   L. L. Haneberg, *Focus Like a Laser Beam: 10 Ways to Do What Matters Most* (San Francisco: Jossy-Bass, 2006), 111–116; L. D. Loukopoulos et al., *The Multitasking Myth: Handling Complexity in Real-World Operations* (Farnham, Surrey: Ashgate Publishing Limited, 2009), 109, 110; S. M. Orsillo, and L. Roemer, *The Mindful Way Through Anxiety* (New York: Guilford Press, 2011), 76–80.

503   Petre, *Father Time*, 52–62.

504   Carr, *Positive Psychology*, 220.

505   Quote Garden, http://1ref.us/8n (accessed February 10, 2010).

506   Seaward, *Managing Stress*, 283, 284, 288,289; E. L. Worthington and M. Scherer, *Psychology of Health* 19, no. 3 (2004): 385–405.

507   K-b. Chan, ed., *Work Stress and Coping Among Professionals* (Leiden: Koninklijke Brill NV, 2007), 48; Seaward, *Managing Stress*, 291–292.

508   Seaward, *Managing Stress*, 219, 220, 230–232.

509   Ibid., 357–369.

510   Ibid., 357, 358.

511   M. S. Bourgeois and E. M. Hickey, *Dementia: From Diagnosis to Management—A Functional Approach* (New York: Taylor & Francis Group, LLC, 2011), 204–206.

512   E. Vasquez, *The Mainstreaming of New Age* (Nampa, ID: Pacific Press Publishing Association, 1998).

513   R. J. Morneau, *A Trip into the Supernatural* (Hagerstown, MD: Review and Herald Publishing Association, 1993).

514   C. R. Holmes, *The Road I Travel: My Journey Along the Narrow Way* (Hagerstown, MD: Review and Herald Publishing Association, 2011), 160–162.

515   Contrada and Baum, *Handbook of Stress*, 102; E. E. Pastorino and S. Doyle-Portillo, *What Is Psychology*, 2nd ed. (Belmont, CA: Thomas Wadsworth, 2009), 559, 560.

516   Contrada & Baum, *Handbook of Stress*, 104–106.

517   Shipton, *Golden River*, 158–198.

518   McMillen and Stern, *None of These Diseases*, 199–201; Pastorino & Doyle-Portillo, *What Is Psychology*, 559, 560.

519   R. F. Paloutzian and C. L. Park, eds., *Handbook of the Psychology of Religion and Spirituality* (New York: Guilford Press, 2005), 482–484.

520   E. G. White, *Steps to Christ*, youth edition (Silver Spring, MD: General Conference of Seventh-day Adventists, 1992), 5–13, 21–25, 35–41, 48, 57–62, 78–85.

521   Carr, *Positive Psychology*, 223; Contrada & Baum, *Handbook of Stress*, 310, 311.

Section III: Spiritual Health

522   *Analects of Confucius*, 6.20, http://1ref.us/ak (accessed April 28, 2015); Quote Garden, http://1ref.us/8n (accessed June 3, 2015); S. Sorajjakool and H. H. Lamberton, eds., *Spirituality, Health, and Wholeness* (New York: Haworth Press, 2004), 37; Thinkexist, http://1ref.us/al (accessed June 4, 2015); Write Spirit Net, http://1ref.us/am (accessed June 4, 2015).

Chapter 11

523   G. E. Veith, Jr., *Postmodern Times: A Christian Guide to Contemporary Thought and Culture* (Wheaton, IL: Crossway Books, 1994), 62.

524   G. Land, *Dialogue* 8, no. 1 (1996): 5–7.

525   A. Oliver, "Postmodern Thought and Adventist Education," 24th International Faith and Learning Seminar, Andrews University, Berrien Springs, Mich., June 20–July 2 (1999): 1–16, http://1ref.us/an (accessed February 10, 2015); Veith, *Postmodern Times*, 43, 44, 58, 59, 73–75; R. E. Webber, *Ancient-Future Faith* (Grand Rapids, MI: Baker Books, 2003), 21–23.

526   R. Jackson and J. Makransky, eds., *Buddhist Theology: Critical Reflections by Contemporary Buddhist Scholars* (London: RoutlegeCurzon, 2003), 215.

527   H. Herrman et al., eds., *Promoting Mental Health: Concepts, Emerging Evidence, Practice* (Geneva, Switzerland: World Health Organization, 2005), 76, 77, http://1ref.us/ao (accessed April 28, 2015).

528   C. Young and C. Koopsen, *Spirituality, Health, and Healing* (Thorofare, NJ: SLACK Incorporated, 2005), 10, 11.

529   National Aeronautics and Space Administration, "What Is the Ultimate Fate of the Universe?" http://1ref.us/aq (accessed February 10, 2015); MarsNews.com, "Terraforming Mars," http://1ref.us/ar (accessed April 28, 2015).

530   Magai and McFadden, *Handbook of Emotion*, 351–354; A. Meier et al., *Spirituality and Health* (Waterloo, Ontario: Wilfrid Laurier University Press, 2005), 16–18.

531   D. Burton, *Buddhism, Knowledge and Liberation: A Philosophical Study* (Burlington, VT: Ashgate Publishing, Ltd, 2004), 2, 14–18, 36.

532   Seventh-day Adventist Philosophy of Education, Policy FE 05, FE 10, http://1ref.us/as (accessed February 10, 2015).

533   Koenig et al., *Handbook of Religion*, 143; Cobb et al., *Oxford Textbook of Spirituality*, 33.

534 Cobb et al., *Oxford Textbook of Spirituality*, 335.

535 Loma Linda University, Medical Center, "Spiritual Health," http://1ref.us/at (accessed February 10, 2015).

536 A. E. McGrath, *Dawkins' God: Genes, Memes, and the Meaning of Life* (Oxford: Blackwell Publishing, 2005), 50, 51.

537 Ibid., 51.

538 J. R. Durant, ed., *Human Origins* (Oxford: Clarendon Press, 1989), 189.

539 P. Davies, *The Goldilocks Enigma: Why is the Universe Just Right for Life?* (New York: Mariner Books, 2008), 222.

540 R. Adler et al., *New Scientist* 164, no. 2218 (2000): 18–25.

541 R. L. Ciochon and J. C. Fleagle, eds., *Primate Evolution and Human Origins* (Piscataway, NJ: Aldine Transaction, 1987), 292–296.

542 K. R. Foster et al., *Trends in Ecology and Evolution* 21, no. 2 (2006): 57–60.

543 Nygren, *Agape and Eros*, 78.

544 E. G. White, *Christ's Object Lessons* (Washington, DC: Review and Herald Publishing Association, 1941), 418–420.

545 Koenig et al., *Handbook of Religion*, 581.

546 K. Hammerås, "The Knights of the Road" (Master diss., University of Troms, 2008), http://1ref.us/au (accessed February 10, 2015).

547 L. C. Madhi et al., eds., *Betwixt & Between: Patterns of Masculine and Feminine Initiation* (La Salle, IL: Open Court, 1987), ix–xv; F. W. Young, *Initiation Ceremonies* (New York: The Bobbs-Merrill Company, Inc., 1965).

548 Madhi et al., *Betwixt & Between*, 44–59.

549 D. P. Ausubel, *Ego Development and the Personality Disorders*, third printing (New York: Grune & Stratton, 1965); C. Wilcox, *Bias: The Unconscious Deceiver* (Bloomington, IN: Xlibris Corporation, 2011), 21–24.

550 Nygren, *Agape and Eros*, 70–75, 104.

551 Ibid., 75–81.

552 Cobb et al., *Oxford Textbook of Spirituality*, 336.

553 Ibid., 119, 121.

554 F. A. Worsley, *Shackleton's Boat Journey* (Kent Town, South Australia: Wakefield Press, 2007).

555 Sorajjakool and Lamberton, *Spirituality*, 7.

556 C. D. Kernig, ed., *Marxism, Communism and Western Society: a Comparative Encyclopedia* (New York: Herder & Herder, 1972), 4: 398–418.

557 McDowell, *Evidence that Demands a Verdict*, 185–189; B. G. Wilkinson, *Truth Triumphant* (Mountain View, CA: Pacific Press Publishing Association, 1944), 31–44, 146–154, 246–267.

558 L. Strobel, *The Case for the Real Jesus* (Grand Rapids, MI: Zondervan, 2007), 101–126.

559 C. G. Starr, *History of the Ancient World*, 2nd ed. (New York: Oxford University Press, 1974), 139–141, 474, 477, 478, 702.

560 T. Cornell and J. Matthews, *Atlas of the Roman World* (Oxford: Phaidon Press, Ltd, 1982), 213, 214; J. B. Doukhan, *Secrets of Daniel* (Hagerstown, MD: Review and Herald Publishing Association, 2000), 105, 106; W. A. Shipton and E. A. Belete, *Visions of*

Turmoil and Eternal Rest (Bloomington, IN: AuthorHouse, 2011), 68–74.

561 Cobb et al., *Oxford Textbook of Spirituality*, 122.

562 A. E. McGrath, *Surprised by Meaning: Science, Faith, and How We Make Sense of Things* (Louisville, KY: Westminster John Knox Press, 2011), 38–40; R. W. Rogers, *The Death of Man as Man* (Bloomington, IN: CrossBooks, 2011), 101–106.

563 L. T. Johnson, *Faith's Freedom: A Classic Spirituality for Contemporary Christians* (Minneapolis: Augsburg Fortress Press, 1990), 78–83.

564 P. Johnson, *Reader's Digest (Australia)* 155, no. 932 (1999): 16–20; R. C. Piper, ed., *Secrets of Happy Living* (Warburton, Victoria: Signs Publishing Company, 1950), 25–29; R. Rice, *Reason and the Contours of Faith* (Riverside, CA: La Sierra University Press, 1991).

565 Rushton, *Altruism*, 2, 3.

566 Seaward, *Managing Stress*, 142–144.

567 McDowell, *Evidence that Demands a Verdict*, 327–359; V. E. Robinson, *Curse of the Cannibals* (Washington, DC: Review and Herald Publishing Association, 1976).

568 N. Jones, *New Scientist* 177, no. 2376 (2003): 14.

569 Sorajjakool and Lamberton, *Spirituality,* 42–47.

570 Herrman et al., *Promoting Mental Health* (2005), 56.

Chapter 12

571 E. Aarvik, The Nobel Peace Prize 1984, Award Ceremony Speech for Desmond Tutu, http://1ref.us/av (accessed April 28, 2015).

572 R. Dawkins, *The Selfish Gene* (London: Granada, 1978), x.

573 Dawkins, *The Selfish Gene,* x; C. Grant, *Altruism and Christian Ethics* (Cambridge: Cambridge University Press, 2001), 6–22, 32–56, 61, 167.

574 F. A. Schaeffer, *Escape from Reason*, book two, in *The Francis A. Schaeffer Trilogy* (Wheaton, IL: Crossway Books, 1990), 231, 232; Grant, *Altruism*, 91–109.

575 F. A. Schaeffer, *He Is There and He Is Not Silent*, book three, in *The Francis A. Schaeffer Trilogy*, 299–301.

576 J. C. Avise and F. J. Ayala, eds., *Arthur M. Sackler Colloquia. In the Light of Evolution. The Human Condition* (Washington, DC: National Academies Press, 2010), 4: 277, 278; A. L. Peterson, *Being Human: Ethics, Environment, and Our Place in the World* (Berkeley: University of California Press, 2001), 193.

577 K. Giselsson, *Grounds for Respect: Particularism, Universalism, and Communal Accountability* (Lanham, MD: Lexington Books, 2012), 117–122; R. A. Mohler, "Is the Sanctity of Human Life an Outmoded Concept?" http://1ref. us/aw (accessed February 10, 2015).

578 Grant, *Altruism*, 183, 188, 189. Schaeffer, *He Is There*, 297, 298.

579 Schaeffer, *Escape from Reason*, 220, 221

580 P. E. Little, *Know Why You Believe*, 4th ed. (Downers Grove, IL: InterVarsity Press, 2000), 144–158.

581 Nygren, *Agape and Eros*, 218.

582 E. Cook, *Journal of the Adventist Theological Society* 18, no. 1 (2007): 64–80; United Nations, "Universal Declaration of Human Rights."

583 Cook, *Journal of the Adventist Theological Society* (2007).

584 Lewis, *Abolition of Man*, 95–121.

585 Cook, *Journal of the Adventist Theological Society* (2007).

586 M. S. DeMoss and J. E. Miller, *Zondervan Dictionary of Bible and Theology Words* (Grand Rapids, MI: Zondervan, 2002); M. L. Morgan and P. E. Gordon, eds., *Cambridge Companion to Modern Jewish Philosophy* (Cambridge: Cambridge University Press, 2007), 200, 201.

587 Cook, *Journal of the Adventist Theological Society* (2007).

588 Grant, *Altruism*, 83.

589 Ibid., 66, 67.

590 Schaeffer, *He Is There*, 291, 292.

591 Ibid., 293–300.

592 E. G. White, *Thoughts from the Mount of Blessing* (Mountain View, CA: Pacific Press Publishing Association, 1956), 77.

593 Nelson, *Outrageous Grace*; Nygren, *Agape and Eros*, 63, 75–81, 104, 132, 133, 146, 147; White, *The Desire of Ages*, 825.

594 Grant, *Altruism*, 188, 189; M. J. Seymour, Sr., *Cultivating Christian Faith* (Bloomington, IN: AuthorHouse, 2004), 157–158; E. G. White, *Steps to Christ* (Washington, DC: Review and Herald Publishing Association, 1908), 37–41.

595 White, *The Desire of Ages*, 504, 505.

596 Ibid., 638.

597 M. Lucado, *A Heart Like Jesus* (Nashville: W. Publishing Group, 2002), 35–39.

598 B. Hybels, *Too Busy to Pray* (Leicester: Inter-Varsity Press, 2001), 56–59.

599 T. A. Davis, *Conscience* (Washington, DC: Review and Herald Publishing Association, 1977), 23–26.

600 Shaffer, *Personality Development*, 432.

601 Wilkinson, *Truth Triumphant*, 23–26.

We invite you to view the complete
selection of titles we publish at:

www.TEACHServices.com

Scan with your mobile
device to go directly
to our website.

Please write or email us your praises, reactions, or
thoughts about this or any other book we publish at:

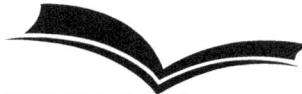

TEACH Services, Inc.

PUBLISHING

www.TEACHServices.com • (800) 367-1844

P.O. Box 954
Ringgold, GA 30736

info@TEACHServices.com

TEACH Services, Inc., titles may be purchased in bulk for
educational, business, fund-raising, or sales promotional use.
For information, please e-mail:

BulkSales@TEACHServices.com

Finally, if you are interested in seeing
your own book in print, please contact us at

publishing@TEACHServices.com

We would be happy to review your manuscript for free.

www.ingramcontent.com/pod-product-compliance
Lightning Source LLC
Chambersburg PA
CBHW080331270326
41927CB00014B/3170